I dedicate this book to my stepfather, Lee, who has built things, fixed things, and helped me with so much over the last 40 years, including hanging bars and building special steps and ramps for my fitness studio to help keep my clients safe.

Thank you!

You will be greatly missed.

TABLE OF CONTENTS

INTRODUCTION

In *Stroke Recovery, Leg Stability, and Walking Gait*, I share illustrations of the many muscles in the body that participate in the movement of the hips, leg, and feet. I discuss different challenges that stroke survivors face, such as drop foot and hyperextended knee. A strong core, back muscles, and posture are extremely important to help the leg, foot, and toes improve in movements. Studies have shown that poor posture can hinder communication for movements between the spinal cord, brain, and movement.

I know that it's tempting for you to skip all the reading and knowledge in this book and just go right to the exercises, **but** I strongly encourage you and/or your caregiver to learn what you can do to help you stay safe and get the best you can out of each exercise.

Gaining knowledge of anatomy and the biomechanics of leg movement can help a stroke survivor understand which exercises will help to improve their walking gait. Often in therapy and exercise programs, people just do the exercises because someone tells them to do so, with no knowledge or understanding of the reason why or how a movement will affect them in everyday life activities.

In many cases, stroke recovery patients do not get enough physical therapy to help them reach their full potential in their recovery. This leaves many stroke survivors seeking help from other sources, such as personal trainers, Pilates teachers, and other professionals in the fitness communities.

As I mention in all my books, I am not a physical therapist. I am a fitness specialist who often meets tibialis stroke survivor clients who have finished their physical therapy and do not know what else they can do or how much further their recovery can go. A stroke survivor's recovery does not end when physical therapy ends.

In the last several years, I have been meeting stroke survivors at much earlier stages in their recovery than I used to. I have always sought out more in-depth and higher education for my training to bring the best care possible to all my clients. The limited physical therapy for many has also forced other fitness professionals, who choose to, to seek out higher education to help bring the best care possible in the guidance for survivors.

Although this book is for stroke survivors and caregivers, it is also a great source for any student needing to learn anatomy for school, physical therapy, fitness, or Pilates and yoga certifications. It is a great take-along to your physical therapist, personal trainers, fitness professionals, massage therapist, acupuncturists, and doctor visits to help you and your professionals work strongly together as a team.

If you have read my other books or watched any of my videos, you may remember me teaching the crucial importance of having a strong core and good posture to help regain balance, stabilization, walking skills, gaits, and arm and leg movements.

Each survivor's recovery, stroke effects, and challenges are different. This is not a step by step following "easy fix" book. Stroke recovery is not an easy fix; It usually requires persistent hard work. This book is a bundle of knowledge with some exercises to help in a stroke survivor's recovery of legs and improving walking gait.

I feel strongly that if we understand our muscles and the movements each muscle performs, it guides one to a better recovery as well as staying injury-free during our daily activities, exercise, and physical therapy programs.

In all my books, I try to keep it simple and to the point, so that it is easier to follow along. As you read through this book, please understand that the muscles are not shared in the exact order that they layer in the body, nor is every muscle listed.

Throughout this book, you will find different exercises and tips that will help you in your recovery. Remember, each stroke survivor has their own stroke effects that they are trying to heal. Not all exercises will apply to everyone.

CHAPTER ONE

MOVEMENTS OF THE HIP AND KNEE JOINTS

The Hip

The hip is a ball and socket joint. These joints allow multidirectional movement and rotation.

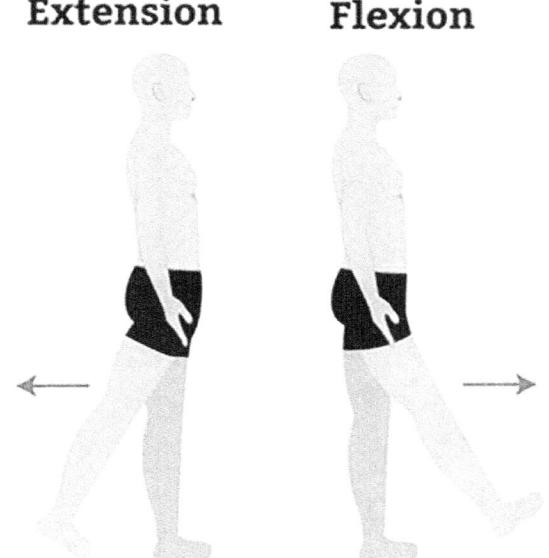

Extension   **Flexion**

Hip flexion and Extension

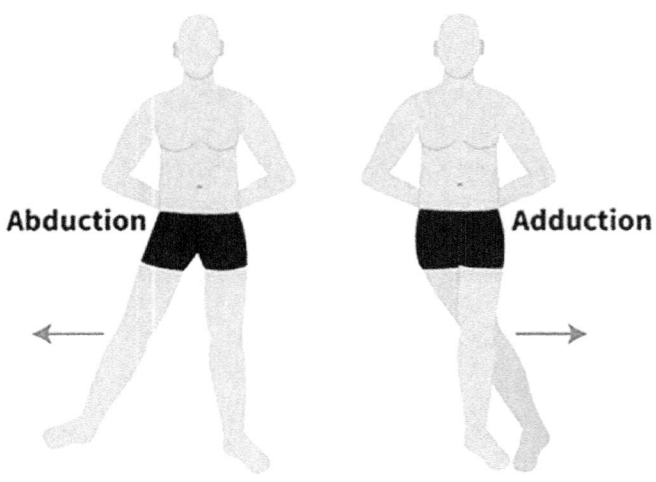

Abduction · **Adduction**

Hip Abduction and Adduction

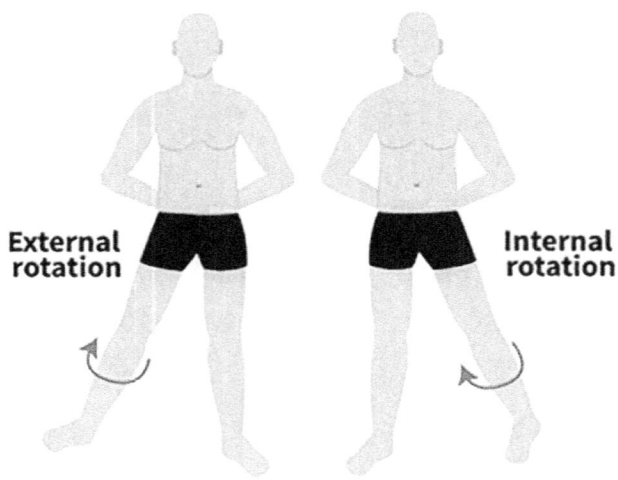

External rotation · **Internal rotation**

Hip External and Internal Rotation

The hip/joint also moves in **circumduction**. This is moving the leg in a circular motion. To perform this circular motion, **it requires flexion, extension, abduction, and adduction of the hip.**

Notice the foot positioning as the hip performs each movement. Stabilizing the core, pelvic, and hips is essential to fix the leg, knee, and foot challenges after a stroke.

The Knee

The knee joint is a hinge joint, and it allows the leg to extend and bend at the knee.

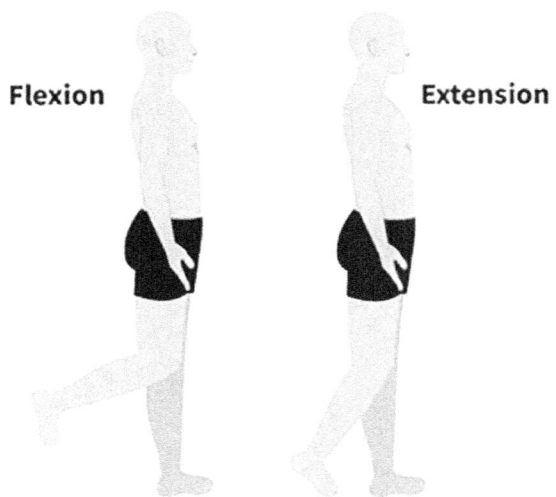

Flexion   **Extension**

Knee Flexion and Extension

CHAPTER TWO

THERE ARE MANY MUSCLES INVOLVED IN WALKING AND STANDING

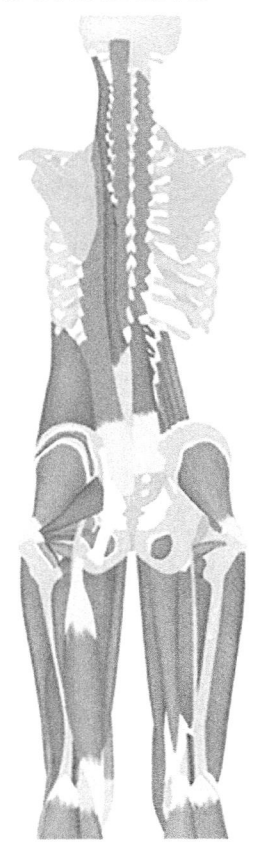

The illustration of the muscles above shows some of the many muscles involved in walking and standing.

The hips, pelvic, and the trunk of the body need to become strong to hold the body upright in the proper posture for the legs and arms to move freely through the many ranges of motions and movements they were made to perform.

As you look at the different hip movements in the illustrations in the previous pages, you can see that if the hips are not stable, these movements will be harder to perform at their full range of motion needed for walking and other everyday activities.

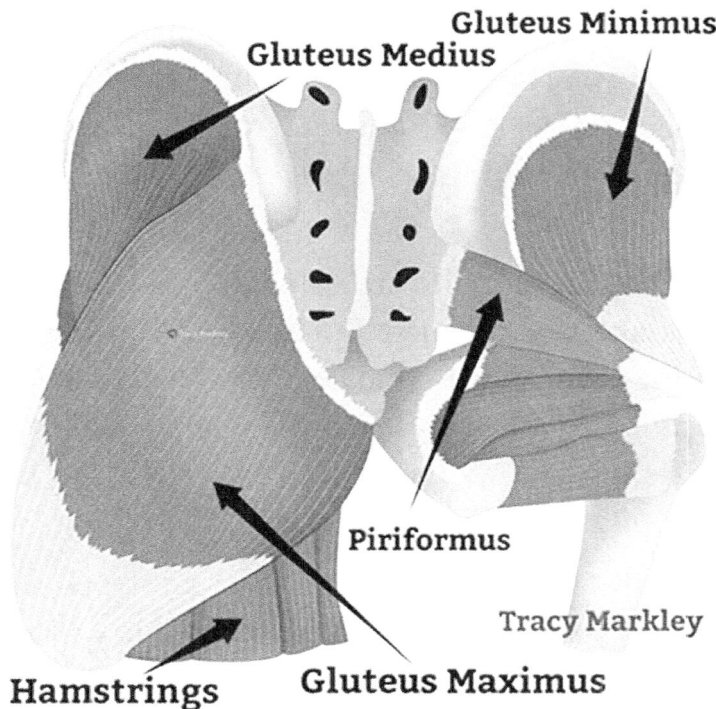

In the gluteus illustration, you will see the large glute muscle and the smaller muscles that are underneath. The large glute muscle extends the femur, which is the backswing of the leg while walking. It also rotates the femur outward. The smaller group of muscles work together to rotate the femur outward. The femur is the large upper leg bone.

We have a **gluteus maximus**, **medius,** and **minimus**. The **gluteus maximus** extends the femur and rotates it outward while the **gluteus medius** and **minimus** abducts and rotates the femur inward.

The glute muscles are immensely powerful. In walking, they complete the backward movement of the step. When someone has "saggy butt," meaning, weak, non-toned, or non-strengthened glutes, this shows that the glute muscles are not performing their primary function in walking.

If the spine and back muscles are weak and there is poor posture, the hips and pelvic will not be strong and stable enough to allow these muscles and other muscles like the **piriformis** and the other hip rotator muscles that you see in this illustration to work properly. This leaves the spine and back muscles to try to assist in these muscles' jobs, leaving the body trying to function and move out of balance, causing pain, weakness, and injury in the back as well as hips, knees, and ankles. Therefore, posture is essential.

As you continue through this book, you will see other muscles involved in walking. Studies show that over 70 percent of the body's muscles are involved in walking.

Gluteus Maximus: Attaches at the ilium and sacrum and to the femur. It extends and rotates the femur outward.

Gluteus Medius: Attaches at the ilium in a twist to the femur. It abducts and rotates the femur inward.

Gluteus Minimus: Attaches at the ilium in a twist to the femur. It abducts and rotates the femur inward.

Piriformis: Attaches at the ischium and the sacrum and to the femur. It rotates the femur outward.

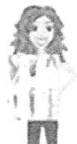 ***Reminders and tips.***

When the hip is rotated out, this is when the foot turns out. Correcting the foot turn out, foot drag, and foot drop begin in the hips.

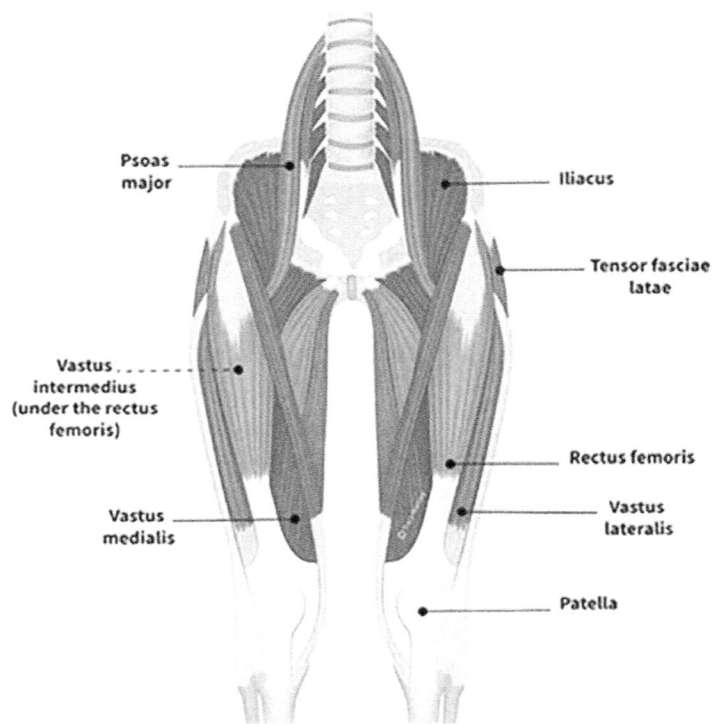

There are four quadriceps muscles. They are the **vastus intermedius, rectus femoris, vastus medialis, and the vastus lateralis.**

They are muscles of the front of the thigh. *The quadriceps help raise and push forward the thigh and leg while walking.*

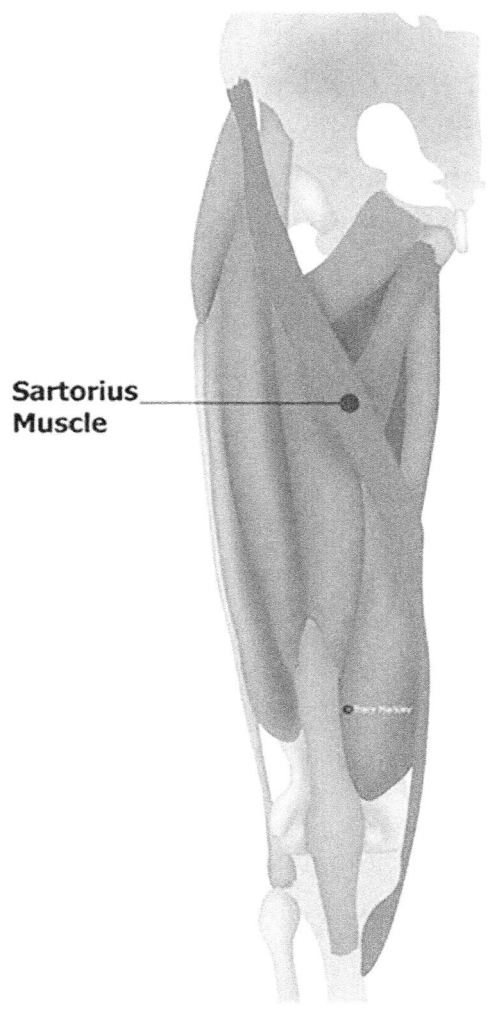

Sartorius Muscle

The **Sartorius** is the longest muscle in the body. It is attached to the front of the ilium, crosses over the medial side of the thigh, and from the knee to the front of the tibia. Although it is an anterior muscle, it inserts into the tibia from behind the knee, and it flexes the foreleg. It also flexes, abducts, and laterally rotates the thigh at the hip. The more survivors, caregivers, and professionals know about the muscles of the body and the movements they perform, the better chance they have in strengthening the body appropriately to help in further and stronger recovery. The **sartorius** helps to lift the leg in taking steps while walking.

Did you know that having any or all these muscles tight or the fascia locked up around these muscles can add to shoulder, hip, knee, foot, and back pain as well as add to movement issues? Remember that the fascia intertwines through the whole body. When fascia is tight, locked up, or stuck (there are many ways to describe it) anywhere in the body it can cause havoc, causing pain and/or limiting movement somewhere else in the body. See *The Spinal Engine and Working Through the Fascia Lines Theories* chapter in this book.

Rectus femoris: Attaches at the ilium and to the tibia through its attachment at the patella. It extends the foreleg.

Vastus intermedius: Attaches to the femur and the tibia through its attachment at the patella. It extends the foreleg.

Vastus medialis: Attaches to the femur and the tibia through its attachment at the patella. It extends the foreleg.

Vastus lateralis: Attaches to the femur and the tibia through its attachment at the patella. It extends the foreleg.

Sartorius: Attaches at the ilium and crosses over the medial side of the thigh behind the knee, then attach at the tibia. It flexes the foreleg. It is also in the group of hip flexor muscles. This is the longest muscle on the body.

Popliteus: Attaches at the femur and the tibia. It flexes the foreleg and rotates it inward. It helps at unlocking the knee so it can flex. The **popliteus** is shown in a later illustration in this book.

Tensor Fasciae Latae: Attaches to the ilium, patella, and tibia. It flexes and abducts the femur.

Tibia: is one of the two lower leg bones. The other is the **Fibula**. The **Tibia** is the larger of these two bones

Fibula: is one of the two lower leg bones. The other is the **Tibia**. The **Fibula** is the thinner of these two bones.

Ilium: is the largest part of the hip bone and the upper part of the hip bone.

Ischium: is the posterior/inferior area of the hip bone. It supports the body while sitting.

Quadriceps: means four heads.

Patella is the kneecap bone.

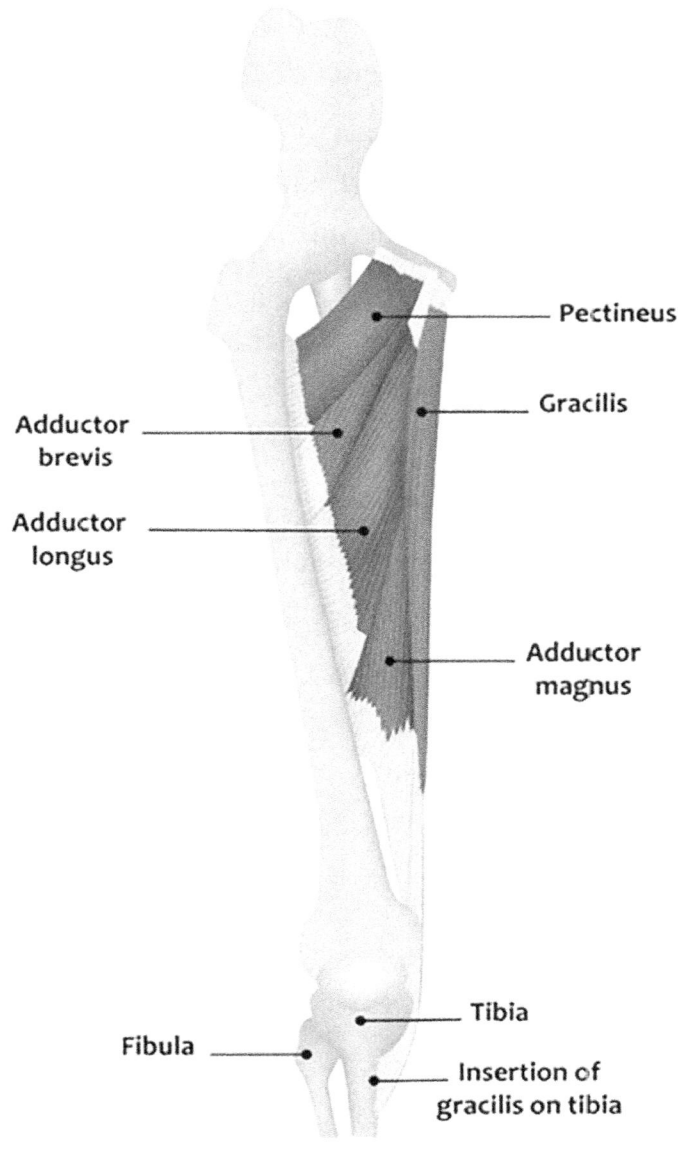

Pectineus attaches to the pubis and to the femur. It flexes the femur.

Gracilis Attaches to the pubic bone and goes behind the knee and then attaches to the front of the tibia. It adducts the hip, flexes the knee, and flexes the foreleg.

Adductor Magnus attaches to the pubis, ischium, and the back of the femur.

Adductor Brevis attaches to the pubis and femur. It adducts the femur.

Adductor Longus attaches to the pubis and the femur. It adducts the femur.

Adductor Minimus (NOT shown in illustration) It attaches to the pubis and the femur and adducts the femur.

All adductor muscles in the thighs pull the legs toward the middle of the body when walking. This helps maintain balance.

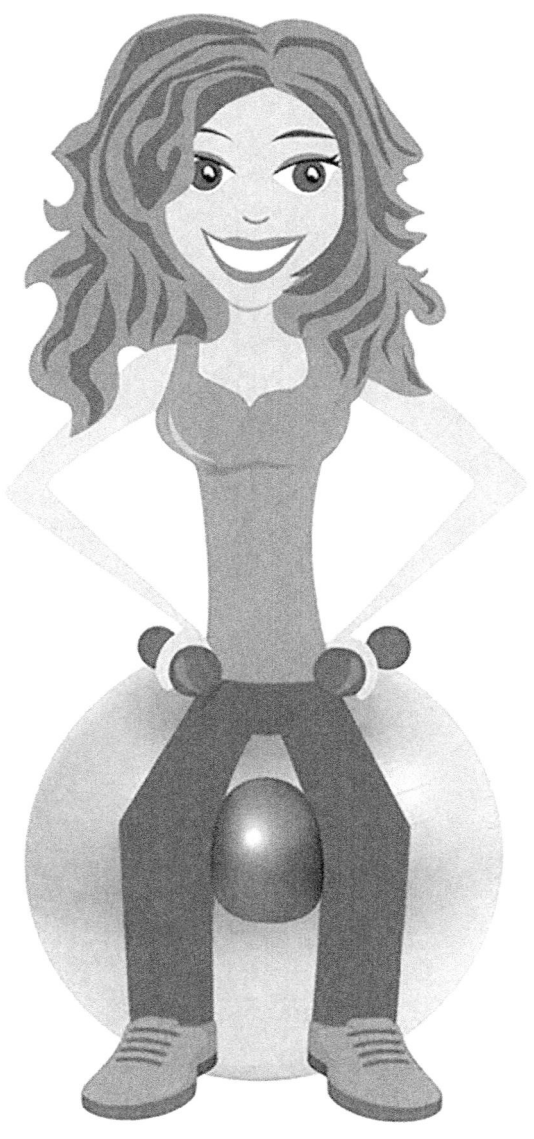

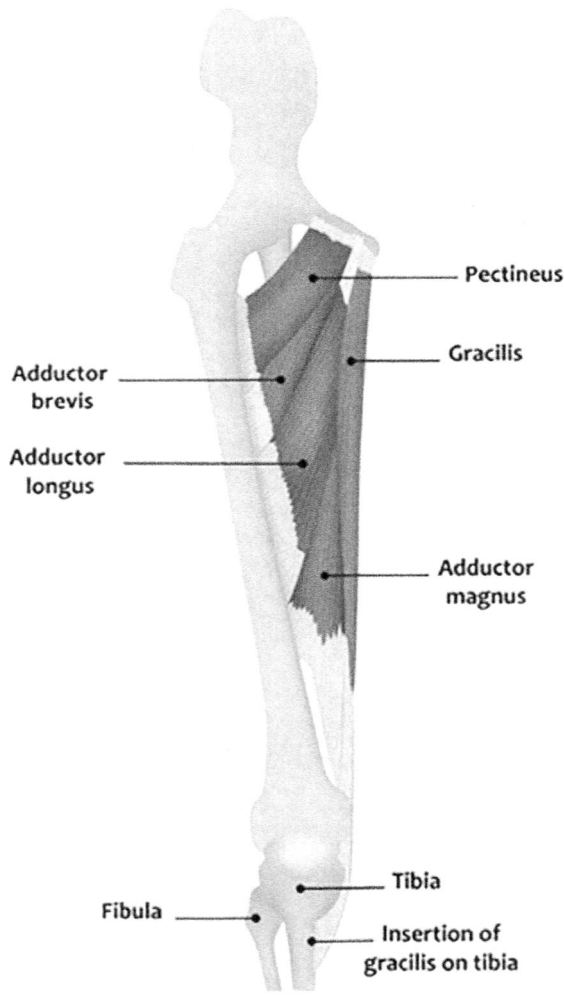

See my books *Tipping Toward Balance, A Fitness Trainer's Guide to Walking*. By Tracy L. Markley, This book includes eight exercises that help with balance and walking.

Stroke Recovery, What Now, <u>When Physical Therapy Ends, But Your Recovery Continues</u>, by Tracy L. Markley. This book includes several exercises for walking, balance, back strength, posture, and stroke recovery.

Hamstrings

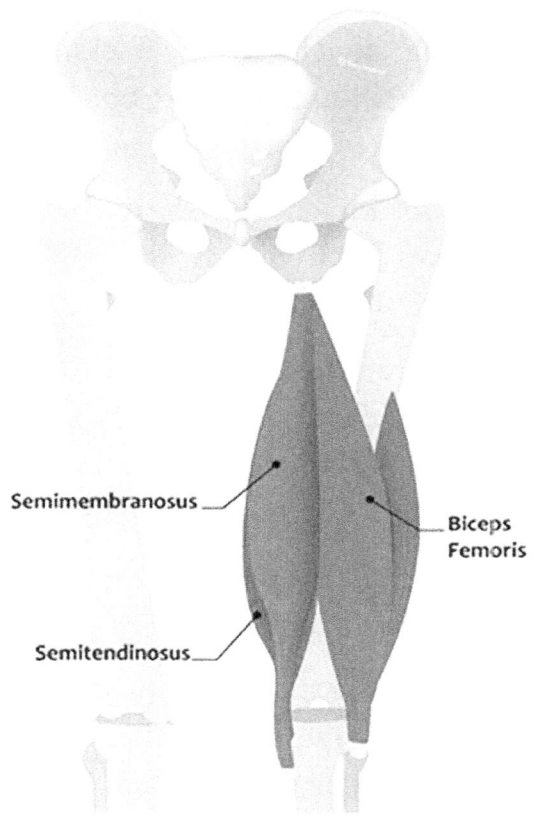

Semimembranosus

Biceps Femoris

Semitendinosus

The hamstrings are on the back of the legs. They move the leg backward in walking steps. When the glutes are weak, the back and/or the hamstrings will try to do the glutes' job. This causes and maintains imbalances and injury. It will limit a stroke survivor's recovery in walking.

Biceps Femoris: This muscle has a *long head* and a *short head*.

Short head: attaches to the back of the femur and the fibula. It flexes the foreleg (lower part of the leg) and rotates the foreleg outward.

Long head: attaches to the ischium and the fibula. It flexes the foreleg (lower part of the leg) and rotates the foreleg outward.

Semimembranosus: Attaches to the ischium and the tibia. It flexes the foreleg (lower part of the leg) and rotates the foreleg inward.

Semitendinosus: Attaches at the ischium and the tibia. It flexes the foreleg (lower part of the leg) and rotates the foreleg inward.

Popliteus: This is a small muscle. It attaches to the femur and the tibia. It flexes the foreleg (lower part of the leg) and internal rotation of the knee joint. This muscle unlocks the knee joint, bringing it from a straight position by helping to bend the leg at the knee joint, which is important for walking.

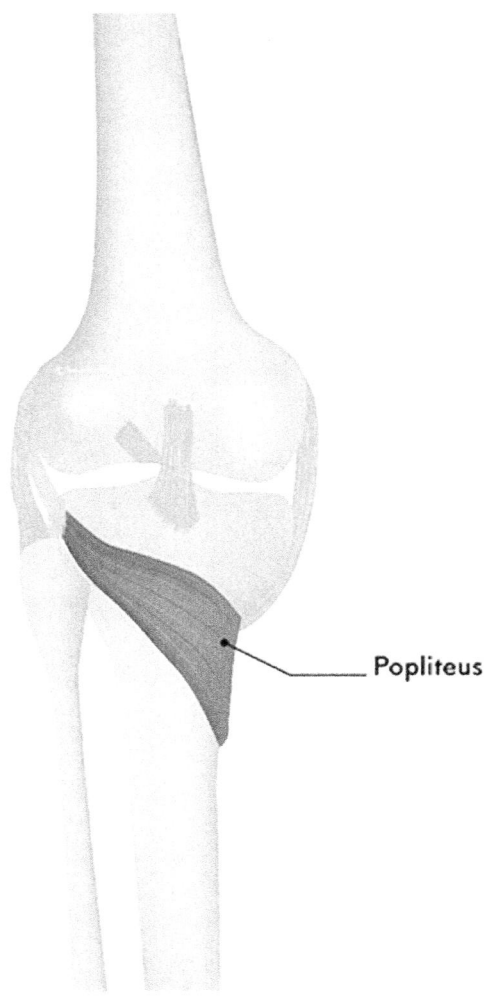

Popliteus

The next chapter will show more of the lower leg muscles and the ankle and foot movements. Also, see the chapters on Knee Hyperextension and Foot Drop.

CHAPTER THREE

HYPEREXTENDED KNEE
AND FOOT DROP

A hyperextended knee is when the knee is pushed past its normal range of motion bypassing the straight position. This can be common for many stroke survivors. The exercises in this book and my videos can help fix a hyperextended knee. **BUT the CORE MUST BE STRONG TO STABILIZE THE PELVIC GIRDLE AND HIPS.** I put that last sentence in bold because if the core is weak, the hips and pelvic girdle will be weak and unstable when sitting and standing. There is less chance that the knee will heal in those circumstances.

If the hips are not positioned properly, the knee cannot be properly positioned to perform the proper movements. I mentioned earlier in the book

Popliteus: Attaches at the femur and the tibia. It flexes the foreleg and rotates it inward. It helps at unlocking the knee so that it can flex. The **popliteus** is shown in a later illustration in this book.

Foot drop is also known as drop foot. I also refer to it as foot drop and leg drag. This is when it is difficult to lift the front part of the foot. The exercises in this book and my videos can help fix foot drop. **BUT THE CORE MUST BE STRONG TO STABILIZE THE PELVIC GIRDLE AND HIPS**. I put that last sentence in bold because if the core is weak, the hips and pelvic girdle will also be weak and unstable when sitting and standing, and the foot drop cannot successfully heal.

Movements that lift the foot off the ground begin in the hips and upper legs, not the foot.

CHAPTER FOUR

THE FOOT AND ANKLE

It is common for stroke survivors to have challenges with walking. One of the challenges is trying to recover things such as drop foot, spasticity, numbness, and more.

Ankle & Foot Flexion

Ankle & Foot Extension

Inversion   **Eversion**

Remember that if you are just performing exercises to work the lower leg muscles to move the foot in these different movements, it will not create the complete movements needed to lift the leg, bend the knee and take a step for walking. The core and trunk of the body must be strong and stable to keep the hips and pelvic in proper alignment. This is essential to support the body so that the muscles that flex and extend the hip, thigh, knee, and foot can perform the movement that takes a step to walk.

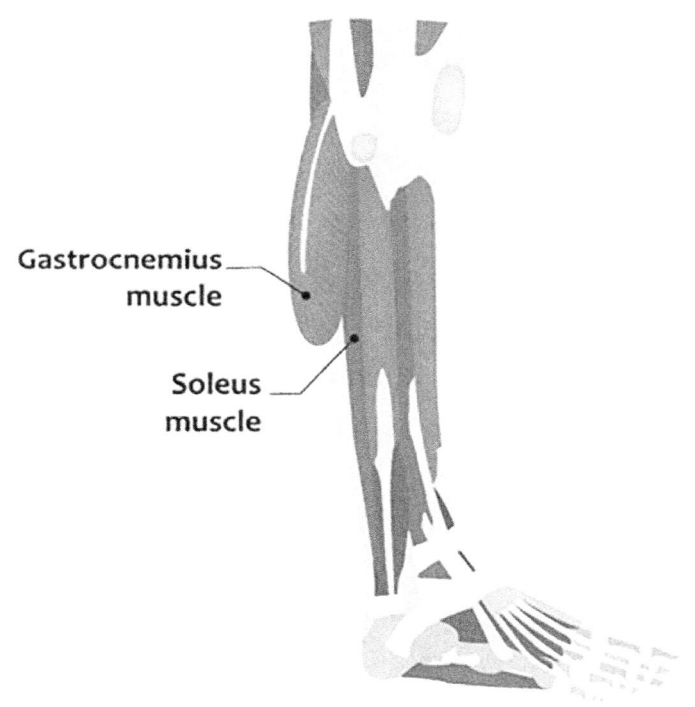

Soleus: Attaches to the back of the tibia and the back of the calcaneus. It extends the ankle and foot.

Gastrocnemius: Attaches to the back of the femur and the back of the calcaneus. It extends the ankle and foot.

Calcaneus: The heel bone.

Malleolus: A bony part on the side of the ankle

Plantaris: Attaches to the back of the femur and the back of the calcaneus. It extends the ankle and foot. This muscle is not labeled in the illustrations in this book.

Flexor Hallucis Longus: Attaches to the back of the fibula and goes behind the ankle and under the foot to the end of the big toe. This toe is known as the toe number one. It extends the ankle and foot. This muscle is not labeled in the illustrations in this book.

Flexor Digitorum Longus: Attaches to the back of the tibia and goes behind the ankle and under the foot to the end of four of the five toes. It <u>does not</u> attach to the big toe. It extends the ankle and foot. This muscle in not labeled in the illustrations in this book.

Tibialis Posterior: Attaches to the back of the tibia and goes behind the **malleolus** and under the foot to the three middle metatarsals. It extends and adducts the foot. This muscle is not labeled in the illustrations in this book.

Peroneus Longus: Attaches to the **fibula** and goes behind the malleolus and under the foot to the base of the big toe. It extends and abducts the foot. This muscle is not labeled in the illustrations in this book.

Peroneus Brevis: Attaches to the fibula and goes behind the malleolus to the base of the pinky toe. It extends and abducts the foot. This muscle is not labeled in the illustrations in this book.

Extension of the ankle and foot is when we stand on our tiptoes. It is also the position when we are sitting down and pointing the toes away from the body.

Flexion of the ankle and foot is when we are standing flat on our feet. It is also positing when we are sitting down, pulling the toes toward the body.

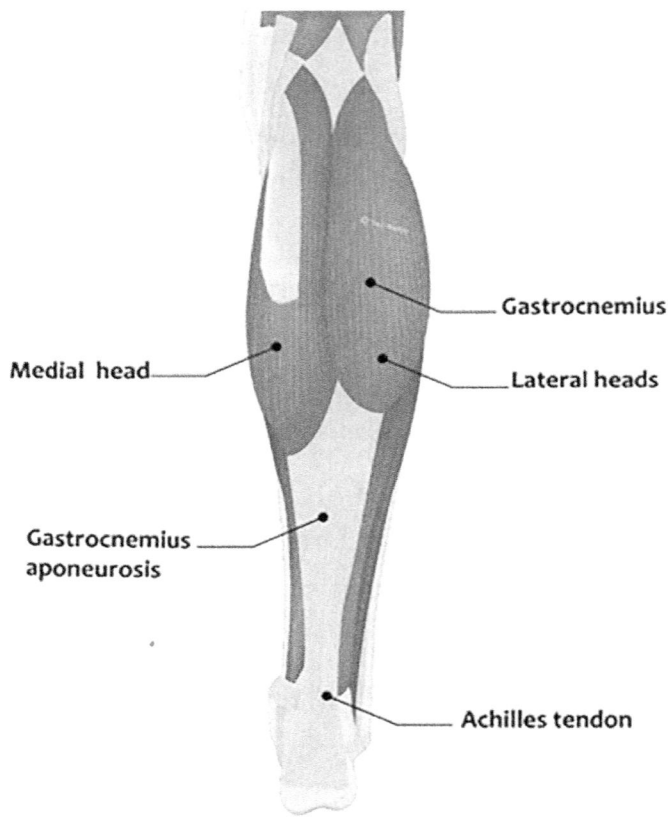

Did you know that having tight calves can add to shoulder, hip, and back pain, as well as movement issues? Remember that the fascia intertwines through the whole body.

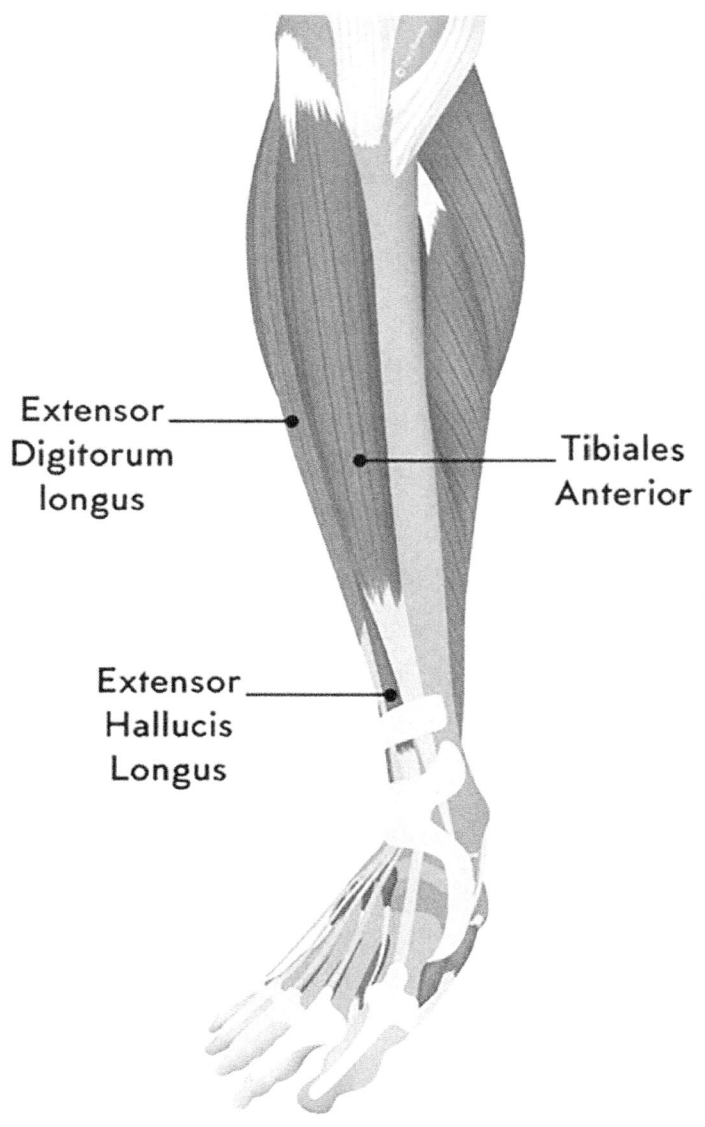

Extensor
Digitorum
longus

Tibiales
Anterior

Extensor
Hallucis
Longus

At the front of the lower leg, there are the tibialis muscles. These raise the foot as one takes a walking stride. The keep the foot up so that it does not scrape the ground in steps. Walking and practicing walking helps keep these muscles strengthened for walking. Not all leg muscles are shown in this illustration.

Tibialis Anterior: Attaches to the front of the tibia and the base of the long bone behind the big toe. This would be the metatarsal number one; it flexes and adducts the ankle and foot. This muscle is not labeled in the illustrations in this book.

Extensor Hallucis Longus: Attaches to front of the fibula and the end of the big toe. It Flexes the Ankle and foot. This muscle is not labeled in the illustrations in this book.

Extensor digitorum Longus: Attaches to the front of the fibula and the ends of the number two to five toes. It **does not** attach to the big toe. It flexes the ankle and foot. This muscle is not labeled in the illustrations in this book.

Peroneus Tertius: Attaches to the fibula and goes in front of the ankle to the base of the long bone above the little toe. It flexes and abducts the ankle and foot.

The reason for sharing all the different muscles is to teach why it can take many different exercises to help recovery the challenges of the leg and foot in walking. Recovery is not a simple list of just a couple of "cookie-cutter" exercises. Any, all, a few, or just one of these muscles can have spasticity and/or the pathways from the brain to the muscles not communicating properly to complete a movement.

Therefore, finding simple answers for exercises to help foot drop and other foot movements after a stroke can be confusing. Every survivor may need something a bit different for them to see progress.

All the muscles just mentioned were only the ones that help extend the foot and ankle. There are just as many on the front of the lower leg that helps flex the foot and ankle.

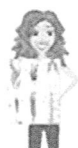

Reminders and tips.

- The calf muscles are commonly known as the **soleus** and **gastrocnemius**. These are among the most heavily used muscles when you take a step, as you can see by the illustrations that there are more muscles involved in the movements that these two muscles perform.

- **While you are doing your therapy and exercises, remember:** Sit down; calf raises isolate the soleus more. Stand up; calf raises isolate the gastrocnemius more.

CHAPTER FIVE

STRENGTHENING THE POSTURAL MUSCLES IS ESSENTIAL FOR STANDING AND WALKING

Posture is essential. These pictures of posture may look familiar to you if you have read my other books. I like to share visuals to help you become aware of your posture when you sit, stand, and walk.

This chapter has a lot of information, and it can be overwhelming for some. As a stroke survivor, you do not have to memorize all the knowledge and muscles. This chapter is here to teach and give visuals and a greater understanding of muscles and movements to help assist you better to a stronger recovery. I feel knowledge is power.

Studies show communication between the spinal cord to both the brain and the limbs can be compromised if the spine or spinal cord is in poor posture. See the pictures of my poor posture. The hip and pelvic girdle cannot be strong and stable to support the leg muscles, which need to gain the strength required to gain a stronger recovery in the legs and walking gait. This includes helping fix foot drop and leg drag. In some survivors, the affected leg feels very heavy, and some have numb spots and no feeling in areas.

When someone stands rounded over with the hips tucked under, as seen in the pictures of me, it limits the range of movement the legs can make in movements such as walking. Poor posture also shows that there are weak core, spine, and back muscles. When this occurs, other muscles try to do the job of these postural muscles, leading to more malfunction.

An important tip while performing your physical therapy and/or training (exercising) on posture, balance, standing, and walking skills is to keep your eyes looking forward. Your body follows your eyeballs. If you look or face down, the body will try to follow. It will keep you in poor posture.

The pelvis's stabilizing muscles must be strong and in balance. These muscles are also essential in walking. You will learn about all these muscles throughout this book.

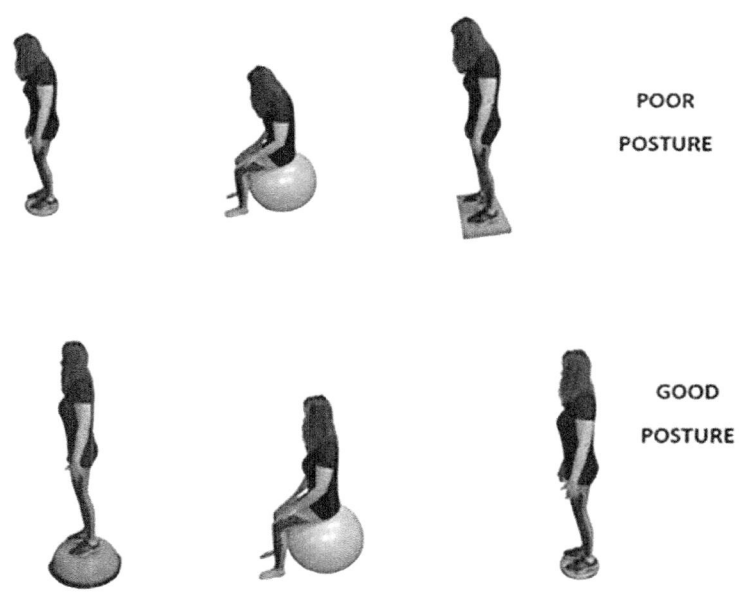

POOR POSTURE

GOOD POSTURE

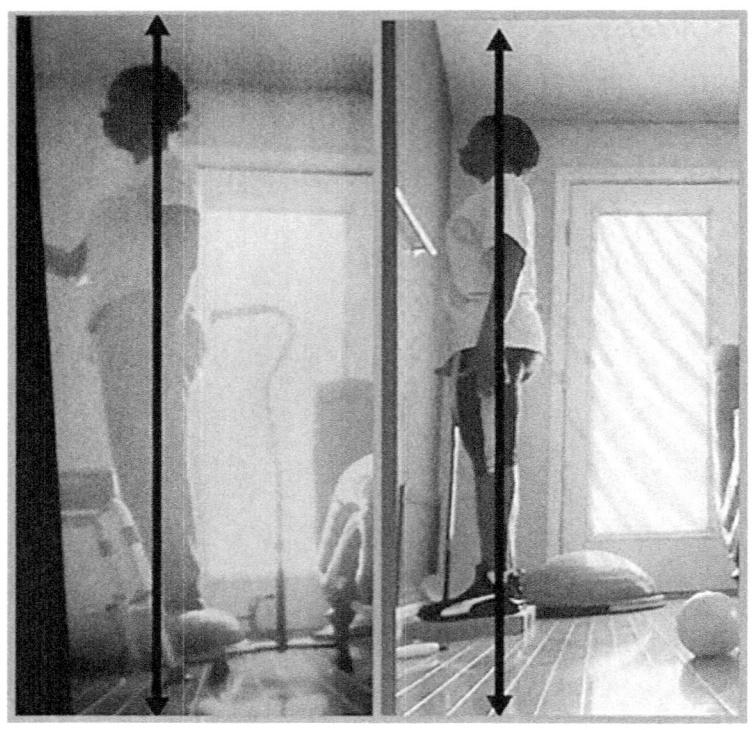

The first picture shows my client leaning slightly forward. This will cause the body to neither rebuild new pathways, the strength, nor the cognitive skills needed to rebuild balance and spatial awareness that is required to be safe in standing, walking, and everyday movements. Also, all the muscles are not building strength in the positions needed to help other muscles also build the strength they need. Studies show that when the body is in proper posture, all the functions and systems work better. In the second picture, she is upright. In this position, the deep spinal muscles can be activated properly to help build the strength and proprioception needed for safer mobility and stabilization in movement.

She is working on her postural muscles and her balance in proper alignment in the second picture. Note: She has a bar on the wall for safety. I suggest always having a bar and a safe environment for your exercising and balancing practices. **Safety First!**

Also, if you look closely at these two pictures, you will see that she is standing on the BOSU® ball in one picture and a balance pad in the other. As you know from my teachings and books, these are both great balance tools when used safely and properly.

In the next four illustrations, I show some of the muscles that will not work to their best performance needed for walking if the body is leaning forward, as seen in the illustration of the man leaning forward to walk.

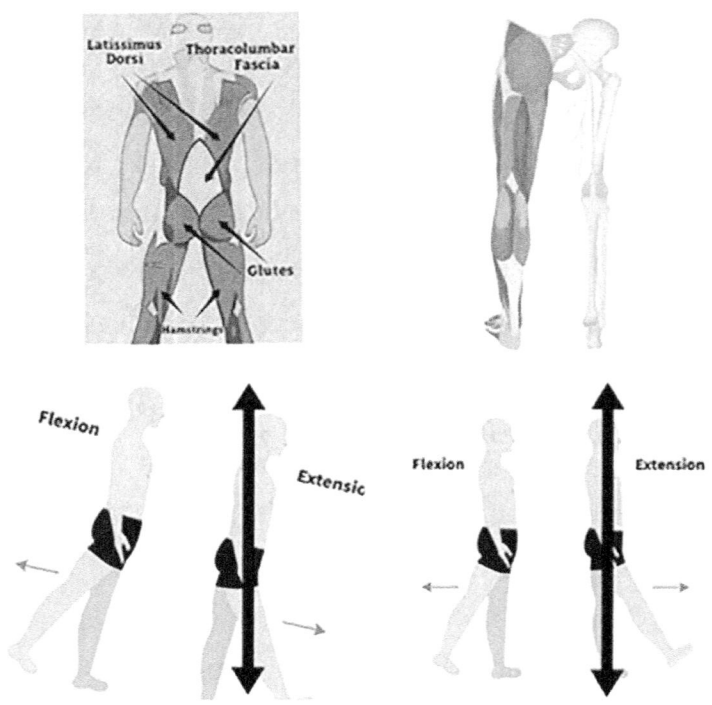

The illustration above is on an extreme angle. This is for teaching purposes to help give a vision of when the body does not line up in proper posture from head to toe, it causes more challenges.

Here is a brief section on some of the core muscles. I also like to refer to them as the postural muscles and the stabilizing system. If you want to learn more about core and spine strength and exercises to strengthen them, see my other books at www.amazon.com/author/tracymarkley.com or www.tracymarkley.com

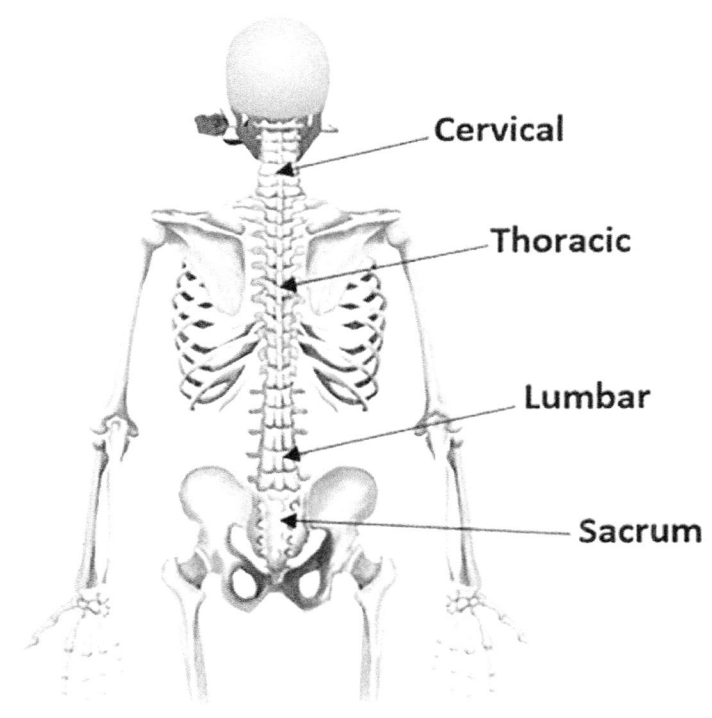

The spine is made up of

7 cervical vertebrae,

12 thoracic vertebrae,

5 lumbar vertebrae.

The sacrum is 5 vertebrae fused together.

At the bottom of the sacrum is the coccyx, which is known as the tail bone (Not visible in this illustration).

The way I remember the number of vertebrae is by something that my college professor taught me.

"We eat breakfast at 7:00, lunch at 12:00 and dinner at 5:00."

If you have read my books, some of what I will share about the **psoas muscle** may sound familiar. The **psoas** is a vital muscle located in the center of the body. It lies deep underneath the transverse abdominal muscle. It is a deep back muscle, and it is the only spinal muscle that directly attaches to the legs. The **psoas** muscle is the only muscle in the back that crosses over the hips and attaches at the front of the body. It attaches to the last thoracic vertebrae and four of the five lumbar vertebrae and at the femur, the upper thigh bone. It is also the bridge between the hips and the back. The **psoas** is often referred to as the **iliopsoas**. This is when the **psoas** and the **iliacus** muscles are being grouped in discussions.

The **psoas** and the **iliacus** are two of the three muscles that help secure the low spine to the pelvis. The **quadratus lumborum** is the third muscle.

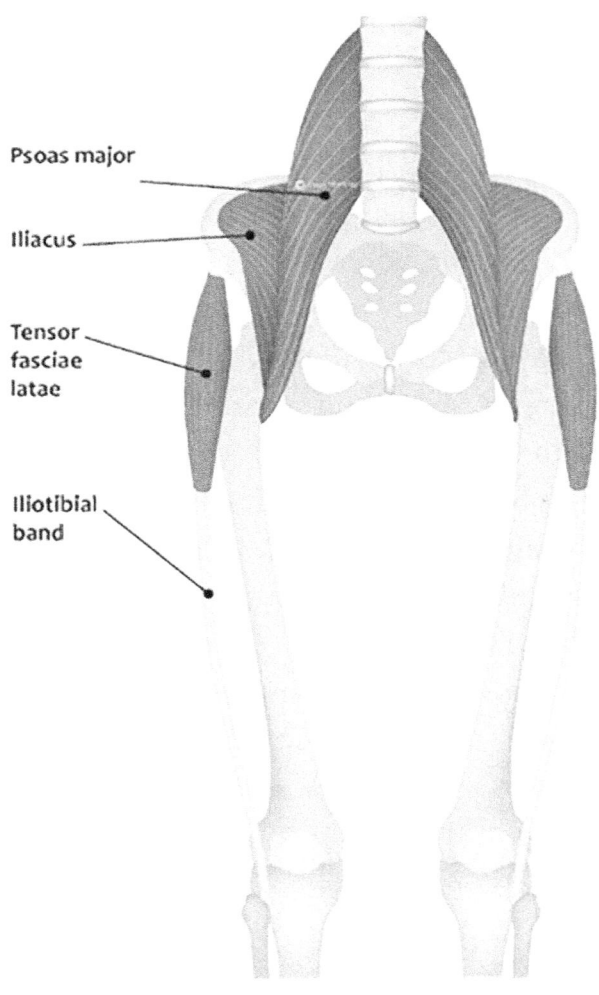

Psoas major

Iliacus

Tensor fasciae latae

Iliotibial band

If the abdominal muscles (part of the core muscles) are weak, the **psoas** tries to perform the work of the abdominal muscles. If the **psoas** is short, weak, and/or tight, it will be difficult to hold the body in an upright position with the shoulders stacked over the hips. Also, there will be more of a challenge for a stroke survivor if the **psoas** has spasticity in any of its fibers. Spasticity does not only happen in the arm and legs. It can occur in any muscle in the body. For example, if there is spasticity in one or some of the **multifidus** or **spinal rotatores,** it could make it more challenging to work on posture, balance, and stabilization of the spine and body. This is another reason to keep working on strengthening the core and postural muscles. See my other books, *Stroke Recovery, What Now? When Physical Therapy Ends, But Your Recovery Continues.* It has a chapter on core and spine muscles plus a chapter on exercises, and the book *The Power of Your Spine, How Back Strength and Posture Pilots the Entire Body.*

Multifidus

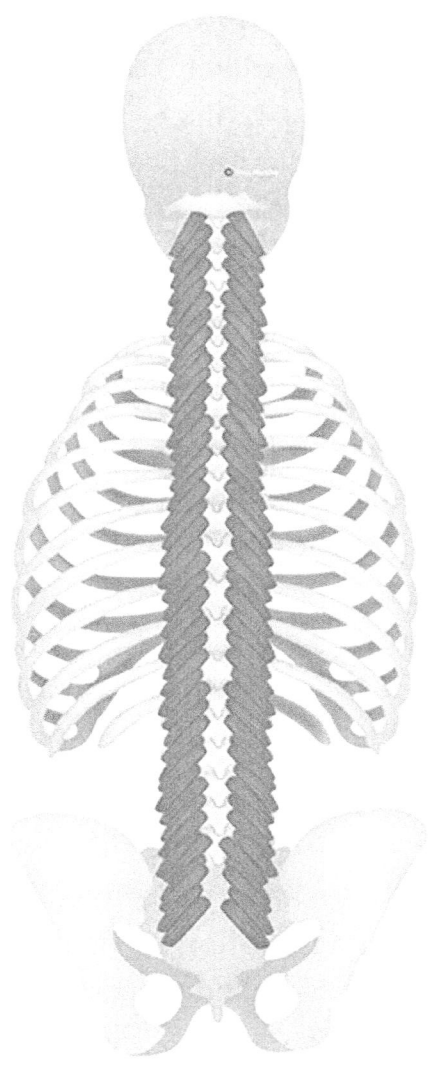

The **multifidus** is a small but powerful muscle. It is the main stabilizing muscle of the spine. This muscle takes the pressure off the vertebral discs so that the body weight can be distributed throughout the spine. If this is weak, you will also have weakness in the low back. The **multifidus** begins to activate before the body moves to protect the spine. It is part of the stabilizing system in the body. The **multifidus** is also one of the muscles in the spine that extends, abducts, adducts, and rotates the spine. To gain a better balance, this muscle must be strong. Performing various exercises combining with the Swiss ball, balance disc, and BOSU® ball will help gain a stronger **multifidus**. Better posture leads to a better balance. See my books, *Tipping Toward Balance or Stroke Recovery What Now?* for exercises on balance and stabilization.

To help this sound simpler, when we bend over from the spine (rounding the spine), the movement is called spinal flexion. When we are moving the spine from flexed position back up to being upright, it is called spinal extension, also known as Axial Extension. Flexion is when a muscle brings two joints together. An extension is taking the two joints farther apart. For example, when we flex our arm to show our arm muscles (the bicep) as in performing a bicep curl exercise, that is flexion. As you extend the arm back out straight, it is an extension.

The small muscles near the vertebrae need to be activated harmoniously. These muscles are postural muscles. Exercising on an unstable surface, such as the Swiss ball, balance disc, and the BOSU® ball stimulates the central nervous system, which are the brain and the spinal cord. It strengthens muscles and ligaments, as well as activating and strengthening all the small muscles along the spinal column.

The **multifidus muscle**, **transverse abdominal muscle**, **diaphragm**, and the **pelvic floor muscles** are all on the same neuromuscular loop. This means it is best if all these muscles are functioning properly; each needs to perform its job individually and as a team. Stated a bit more complicated, it means a sequential segmental neuromuscular stimulation with closed-loop feedback. If the transverse muscle is weak, the pelvic floor, the multifidus, and the diaphragm cannot gain proper strength to perform their jobs in a healthy, functioning body.

Often stroke survivors need to strengthen and correct their posture. Even for seniors and others with balance and stabilization issues, gaining strong postural muscles is essential. Proper posture must be strengthened to help the other stabilizing muscles to hold the body strongly upright so it can achieve a posture in which the shoulders are stacked over the hips. If the head is upright and balanced over the shoulders, we have a better balance. The stability in the pelvis and hips must be made so that the lower limbs and joints can gain strength, function in alignment, and perform properly for safe movements.

Transverse Abdominal Muscle

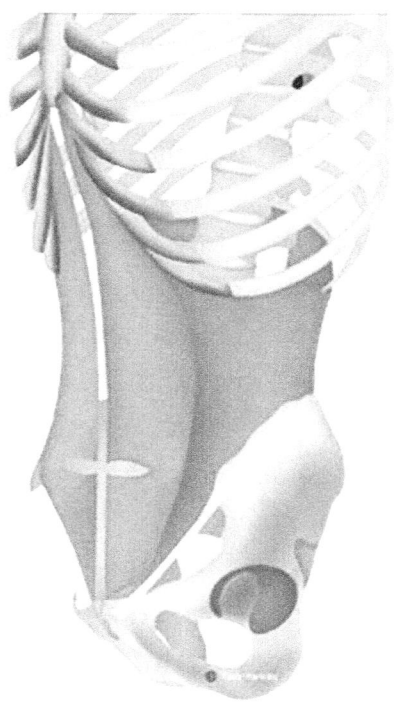

The **transverse muscle** is the deepest of the abdominal muscles. This is not a spine or back muscle, but if this muscle is not strong, the **multifidus spine muscle** cannot be strong. The **transverse muscle's** critical function is to stabilize the lower back and pelvis before movement. It is the deepest abdominal muscle, wrapping around the body to act like a corset. It helps stabilize the hips and pelvic. When engaged, it also pulls the belly in and provides support to the **thoracolumbar fascia**. It is the stabilizer of the shoulder girdle, the head, neck, pelvis, and lower extremities.

For those who are trying to correct posture or are in rehabilitation to learn to stand and walk again or someone who has rounded shoulders and poor posture, it is essential to strengthen this muscle. It must be strengthened to help the other stabilizing muscles to hold the body strongly upright so that it can achieve a posture in which the shoulders are stacked over the hips. If the head is upright and balanced over the shoulders, we have a better balance. The stability in the pelvis and hips must be made so that the lower limbs and joints can gain strength, function in alignment, and perform properly for safe movements.

Before we move forward to another muscle, I hope it is becoming clearer to you just how muscles work together to help other muscles in the body perform their jobs.

The **pelvic floor** muscles work as stabilizers of the abdominal and pelvic organs. The pelvic floor muscles and the gluteus (buttock) muscles are made to work and move in opposite directions.

One must be able to engage the pelvic floor without engaging the gluteus muscles to obtain optimal core strength. These two muscles must be separated in the brain and nervous system for overall body functioning. This also plays a role in preventing back issues. The transverse muscle must be strong for the pelvic floor to become strong and function properly since they are on the same neuromuscular loop.

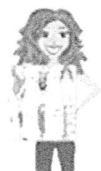 ***Reminders and tips.***

In each one of my books, I share this in the anatomy section:

The **transverse abdominal muscle**, the **multifidus muscle**, **diaphragm**, and the **pelvic floor muscles** are all on the same neuromuscular loop. This means it is best if all these muscles are functioning properly; each needs to perform its job individually <u>and</u> as a team. If the **transverse** muscle is weak, the **pelvic floor**, the **multifidus**, and the **diaphragm** cannot gain proper strength to perform their jobs for a healthy, functioning body.

The Other Abdominal Muscles

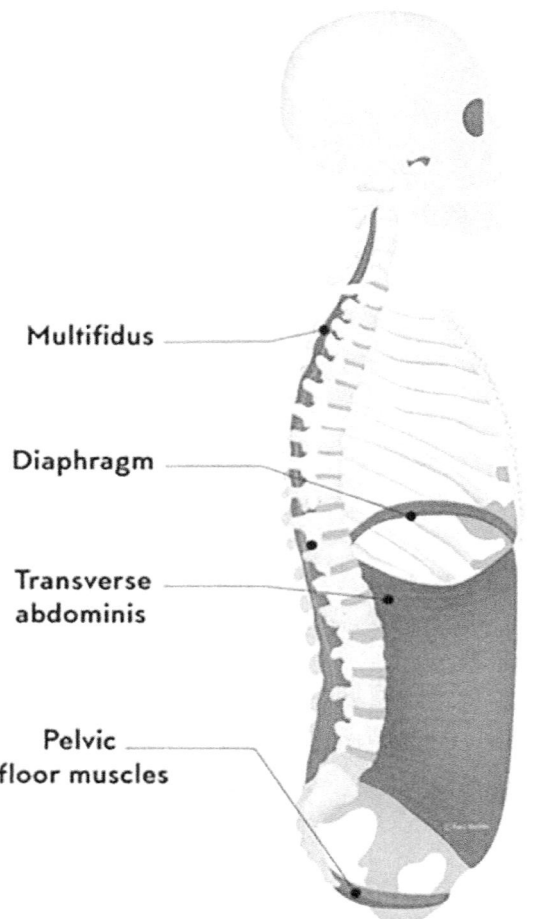

The **transverse abdominals** were mentioned earlier in the book. Now let us look at the other three abdominal muscles.

Rectus Abdominus

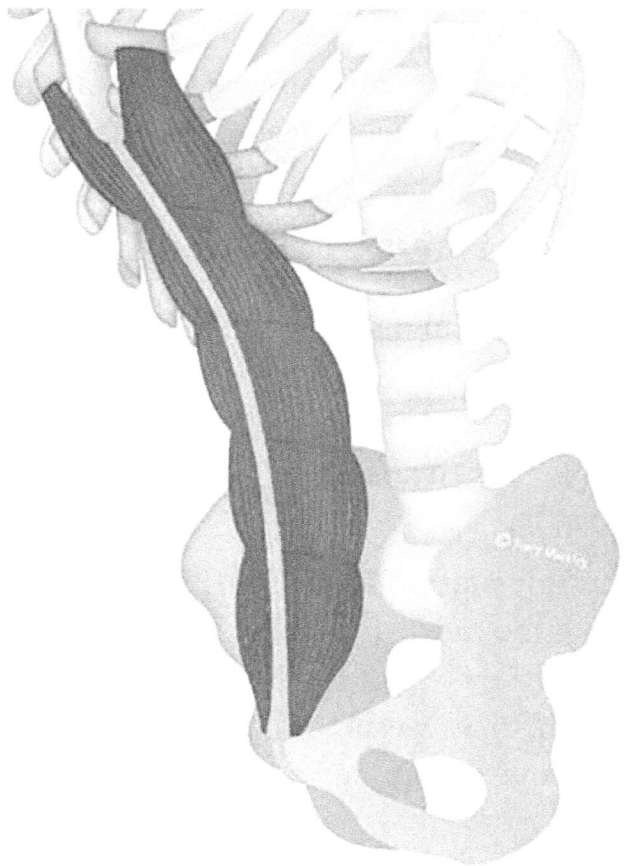

The **rectus abdominus** is the most superficial abdominal muscle. This is the muscle that creates the "six-pack" appearance. It attaches at the front of the ribs 5 through 7 and to the pubis. It flexes and adducts the spine. It enables the tilt of the pelvis and the curvature of the low spine. It also adducts the ribs causing exhalation. Often when people just do abdominal crunches and no real functional training of the abs and core, this muscle can get tight, adding or causing back pain.

Internal Oblique

The word oblique, according to the *Oxford Dictionary*, means neither parallel nor a right angle to a line, but slanting at an angle. Both the **internal** and **external oblique** muscle fibers run on an angle.

The **internal oblique** is on the lateral (side) aspect of the trunk. It attaches at ribs 10 through 12 and to the crest of the ilium (pelvic bone). It adducts the ribs, causing exhalation. It also flexes, abducts, and adducts and rotates the spine.

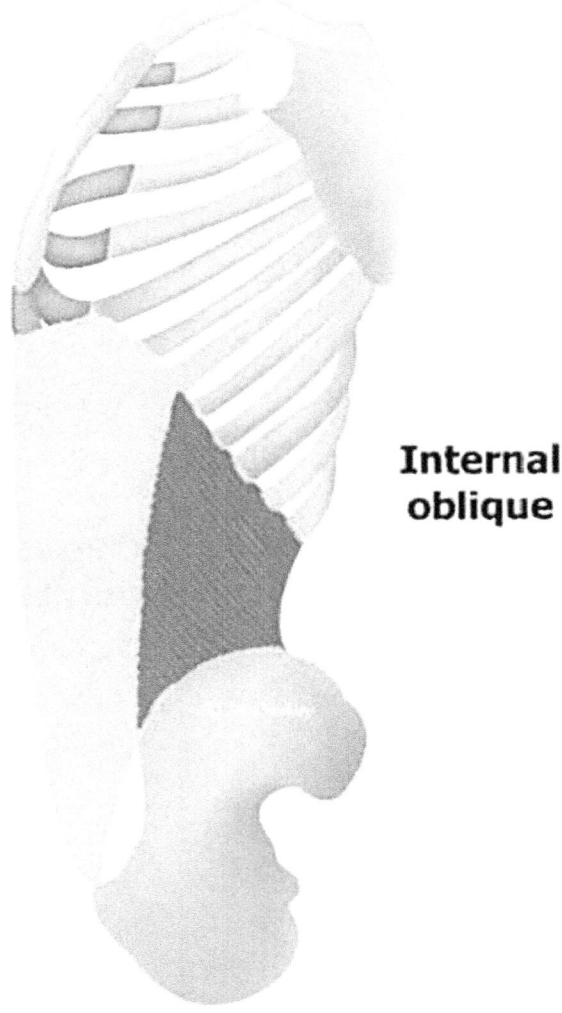

Internal oblique

External Oblique

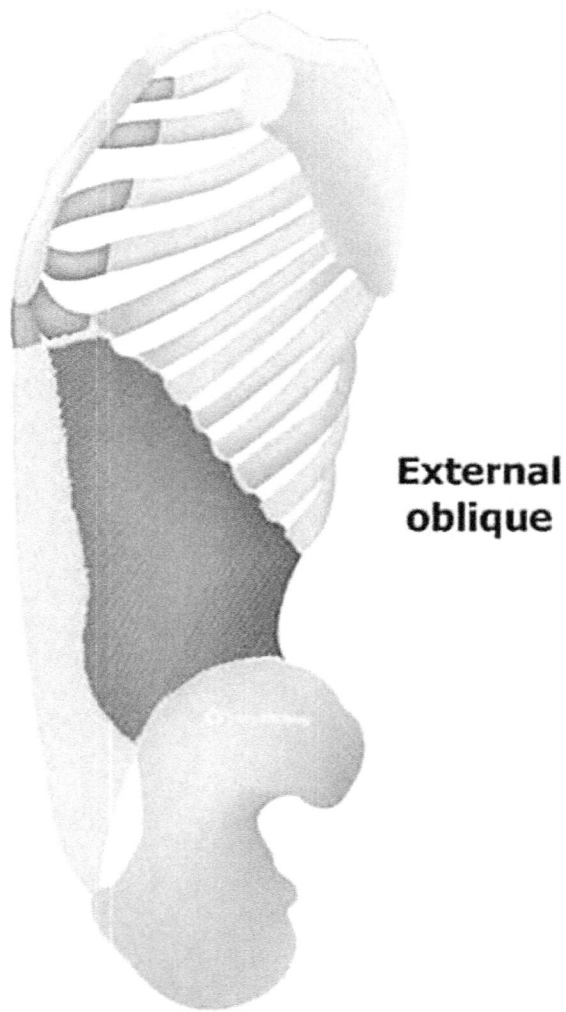

External oblique

The **external oblique** attaches from rib 5 through 12 and to the crest of the ilium. It adducts the ribs, causing exhalation and flexes, adducts, and rotates the spine.

If the deep spine muscles that you read about earlier in this book are weak and not performing their job properly, these outer muscles will pull harder on the spine, which can lead to injury and malfunction. It is especially important to strengthen the body from the inside out, just like a baby develops. This is a key to balance, spine and back care, proprioception, stabilization, and protection of the spine. It is also the key to building all the spine and core muscles to their best strength so all the muscles can focus on only the job they were made to do. This also leaves the body less fatigued.

Abdominal muscles contract with each step when we walk.

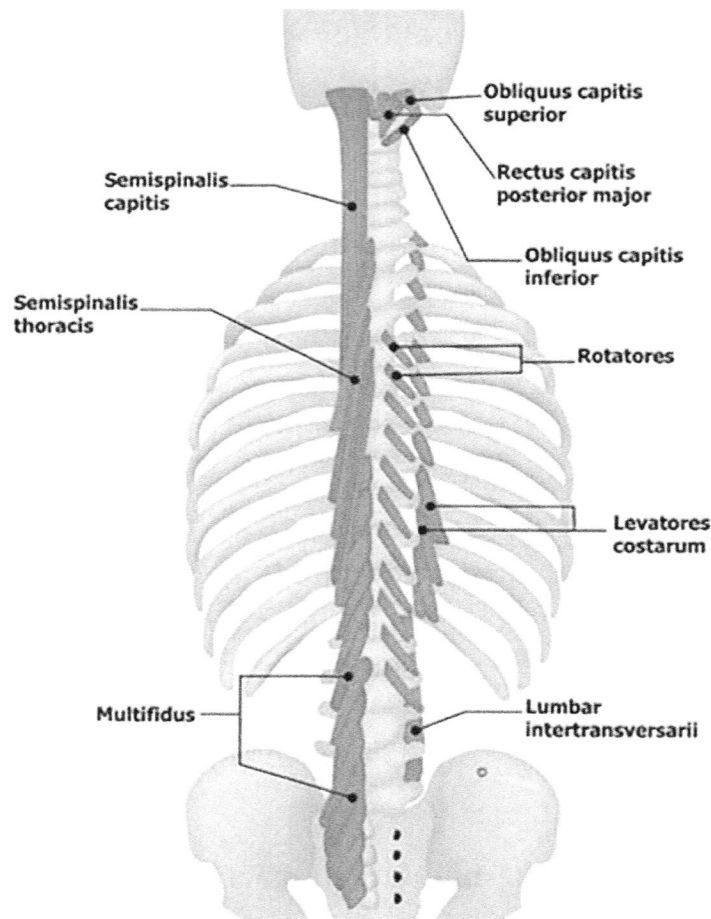

In the illustration above, the right side shows sections only for learning purposes. They are not drawn to their full attachments throughout the whole spine.

The **Transversospinalis group** consists of:

The **rotators**, **interspinales**, and **intertransversarii**.

These muscles are essential for providing proprioception feedback between the brain, back, and entire body.

Rotators - The job of these muscles is to extend the spine and rotation to the opposite side. It moves with proprioception, bringing balance when the body is in movement. They are the deepest and most medial layer of spinal fascial. They extend the spine and rotation to the opposite side. This group of muscles has a lot to do with proprioception, especially the rotators and the **interspinales**. The **interspinales** has a lot to do with the feedback between the back and brain and from the brain to the back. They are the deepest (deeper than the multifidus) and have the most medial layer of spinal fascia. "Medial" means it is the closest to the middle of the body.

Interspinales – Move the spine in segmental extension. This muscle brings a lot of proprioception for the back, balance, and stability of the spine and body in movement.

Intertransversarii – Moves the spine in small segmental motions and lateral flexion of the spine.

They are small muscles that are on both sides of the spine.

The **Interspinales** and **Intertransversarii** muscles move and stabilize the spine. They also play an important role in body awareness and proprioception.

Therefore, it is so important to strengthen the core and spine from the inside out. The body communicates from movement and moves, starting deep in the spine. This is why when I train clients to regain their ability and cognitive skills, such as balance, spatial awareness, and proprioception, I begin with simple but extremely effective exercises like standing on balance discs, balance pads, and/or BOSU® balls. This helps rebuild these muscles and their natural communication to the brain and back.

Quadratus Lumborum

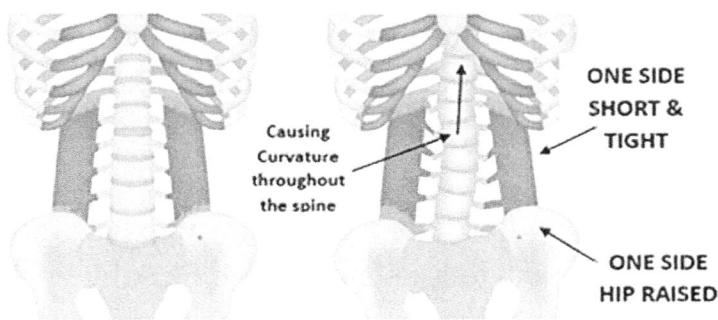

Causing Curvature throughout the spine

ONE SIDE
SHORT &
TIGHT

ONE SIDE
HIP RAISED

The **quadratus lumborum (QL)** (as you can see in the illustrations) attaches from the lumbar vertebrae and rib 12 to the crest of the ilium. It stabilizes the pelvis (hip girdle) when walking and laterally flexes the spine. It has three layers of fibers that move in three different directions. The quadratus lumborum can cause a lot of pain. When this muscle is only activated (or in spasticity) on one side, the trunk is bent towards that direction. The **QL** is one of the muscles that help secure the low spine to the pelvis.

As you can see in the illustration of the **quadratus lumborum**, the one the right shows that if one side of the **QT** is shorter than the other side, it can hike up the pelvis/hips. This will affect the whole body. It can affect shoulder joint and arm movements also.

When someone sits with their hips off to one side, this imbalance will happen to other deep muscles of the spine as well. This includes the **psoas** muscle.

For example, if someone is trying to learn to walk again, and they spend much time sitting with the muscles in this position. When they stand or walk, they will not have the strength, balance, and muscle connection to regain the skill at their best. These illustrations are also another visual to show the power of the spine muscles.

The clients who work on their posture everywhere they go, not just when they are with me, get the best results.

Here is an example of a client who is learning to walk again after a stroke. In the first picture, you can see how his hips are off to one side, and his posture is poor. When he tries to stand up from that position, it does not work. He is attempting to begin standing up from sitting to standing in a **faulty and weak functional position**.

In the second picture, you can see how his hips, legs, knees, and feet are in a good position to move from sitting to standing. It may not be easy to see in these photos, but I had him change his sitting cushion in his wheelchair. In the first picture, he is sitting on a cushion that has no support for his hips and spine, and he just sank into it. In the second picture, he is sitting on a cushion that is made to give his hip and spine support in computer chairs. Switching the seat cushions greatly helped him to maintain a proper seating position needed to aid the functional movement needed to stand and walk. **Be aware of the posture your hips and pelvic are in before you stand up.**

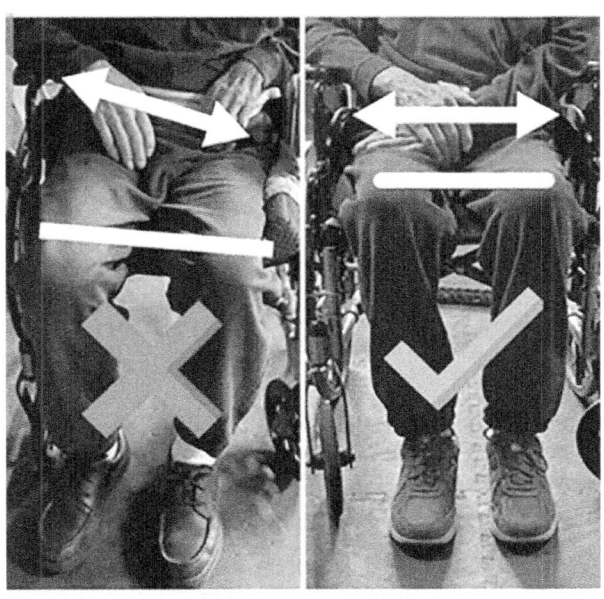

Next, you will see several illustrations to help you understand how the muscles and spine connect. FYI, the sciatica nerve comes through the 4th and 5th lumbar vertebrae. You will see some of the illustrations are on angles as well to help have a visual to what is going on with the muscles when we are in a poor posture as we sit and stand. The goal is to strengthen both sides of the evenly for safer and stronger movements in everyday life and what is needed for safe walking.

How can the many leg muscles that attach at the pelvic bones get the chance to become strong in balance if the pelvic position and posture are crooked? See leg muscle illustrations and their attachments throughout this book.

The core of the body needs to become strong to help bring the hips and pelvis to be stable and in proper alignment.

The position the body spends more time in is usually the position the body will try to use for everyday movements such as the example in the previous pictures. If a person sits for hours a day in a poor spine and hip position, the body will try to use that position for all activities, and the communication between the brain and spinal cord can be compromised. If he sits upright in good posture with his hips positioned properly, the body will be stronger to move properly when needed as well as the communication between the spinal cord and brain will be better.

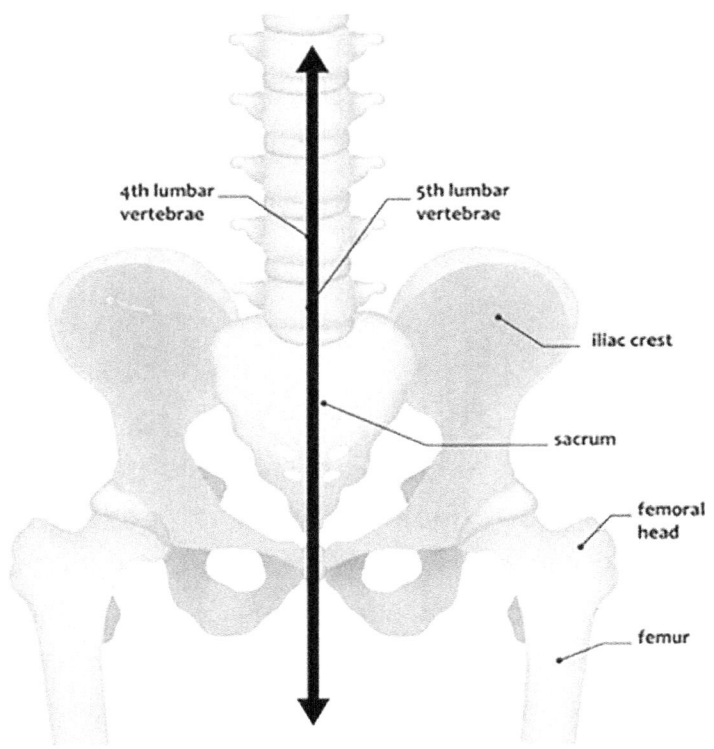

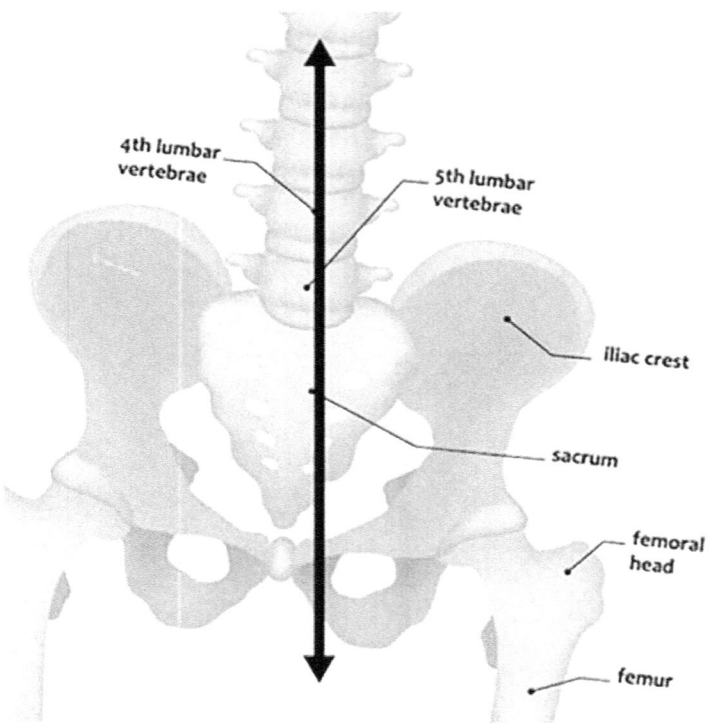

4th lumbar vertebrae

5th lumbar vertebrae

iliac crest

sacrum

femoral head

femur

The next few illustrations were purposely placed in this book on extreme angles for teaching purposes to help you understand that many of the deep and surface muscles throughout the core and legs will not line up in balance to function properly for movements. **This leaves the brain to try to rewire and heal (neuroplasticity) in malfunctioning positions**.

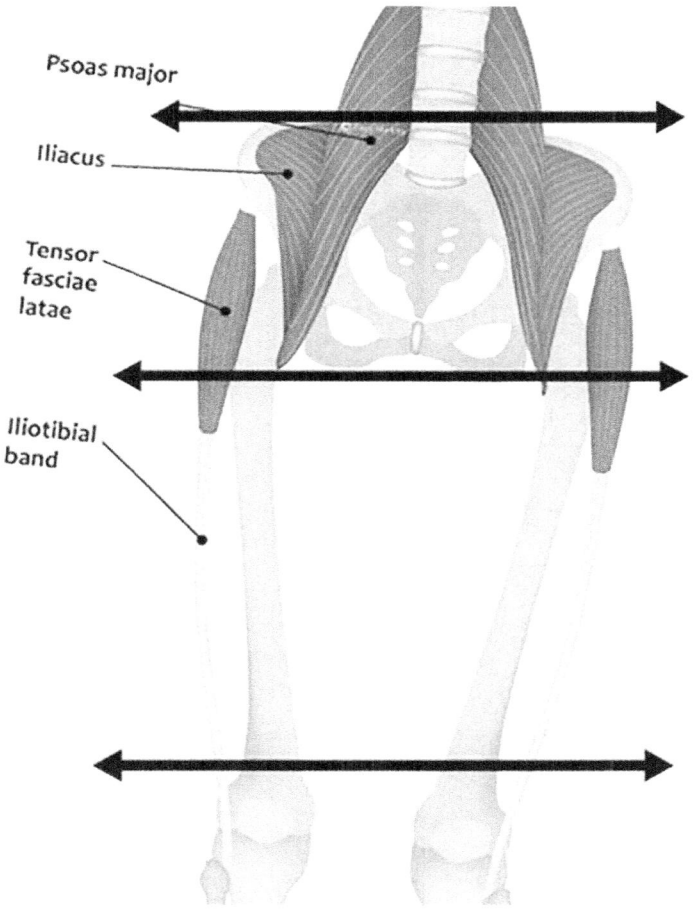

Psoas major

Iliacus

Tensor fasciae latae

Iliotibial band

When the pelvic is weak, tight, imbalanced, and crooked, it maintains the muscles, joints, and movements below to be misaligned and not perform properly.

This is a big issue in foot drop.

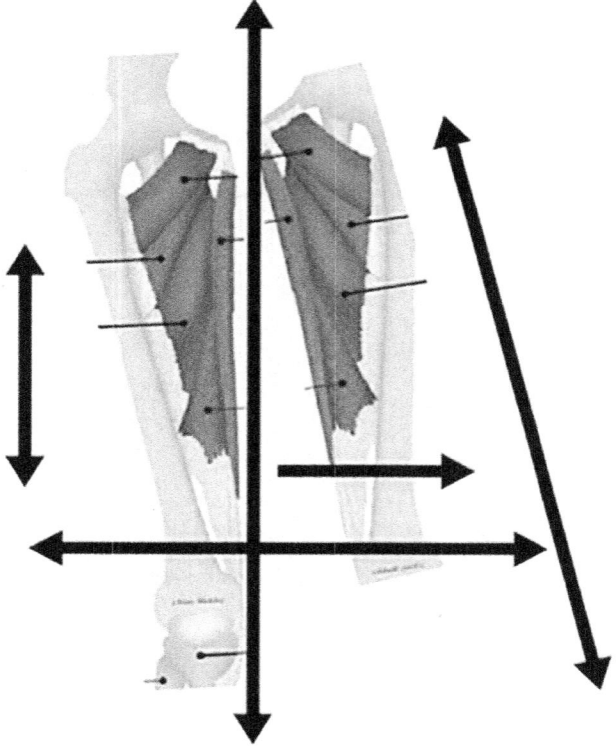

The illustration above shows the position of hips and legs with most people who have drop foot and or foot drag. These inner thigh muscles attach at the pelvis and the femur (upper thigh bone).

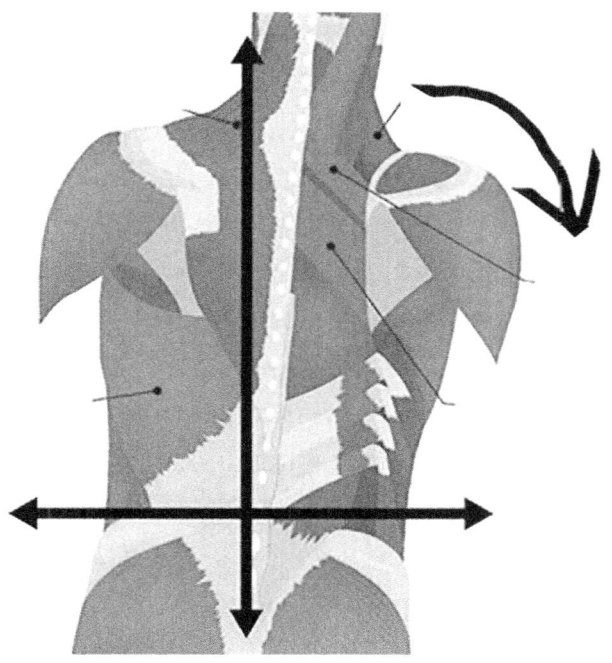

When the pelvis is crooked, the muscles above CANNOT become balanced in strength to help the whole body move smoothly in movements, such as locomotion, which is needed for a healthy and safe walking gait. Usually, the spine becomes crooked, but for teaching purposes, that is not shown in these illustrations.

Each muscle on either side of the spine remains uneven and unbalanced between both sides. This causes the muscles not to be able to work in synergy with the opposite side. The muscles end up shorter and tighter on one side of the spine and cause uneven hips, knees, and shoulder joints. The arms cannot swing evenly, or the hips rotate evenly for a strong walking gait. Although in many cases, the stroke-affected side's arm is having challenges in movement as well, but not always. Some survivors' only challenge left physically for recovery is the foot and walking gait. As a reminder, always take the suggestions in this book, and all my books, to how it can relate to your case. All survivors are different, and each person's recovery is in different phases and time frames.

According to the Webster dictionary, the word **locomotion** means *to move at a regular pace by lifting and setting down each foot in turn, never having both feet on the ground at once.* According to Merrian-Webster dictionary, the medical definition of **locomotion** is *an act or power of moving from place to place and progressive movement.*

As years of studies have been made, the perceived walking movement shows as just the function of the legs being the main movements for walking, however, it has been proven that the spine and the core are the main engines for locomotion. See the chapter "The Spinal Engine and Working Through the Fascial Lines Theories."

I think by now, as you read through this book, and if you have seen my other books, it should make sense as to why getting the core and spine strong is crucial.

CHAPTER SIX

THE SPINAL ENGINE AND WORKING THROUGH THE FASCIA LINES THEORIES

The Spinal Engine Theory

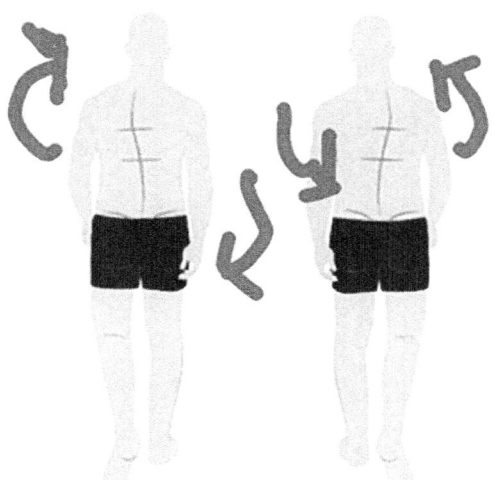

A bove, you will see that when the left arm swings forward, the upper spine rotates forward on the left as the right hip rotates back as the spine rotates for walking steps. This follows the ***Spinal Engine Theory***, which I believe is the correct theory. The spine rotates as we walk.

Latissimus Dorsi
Often referred to as the "Lats."

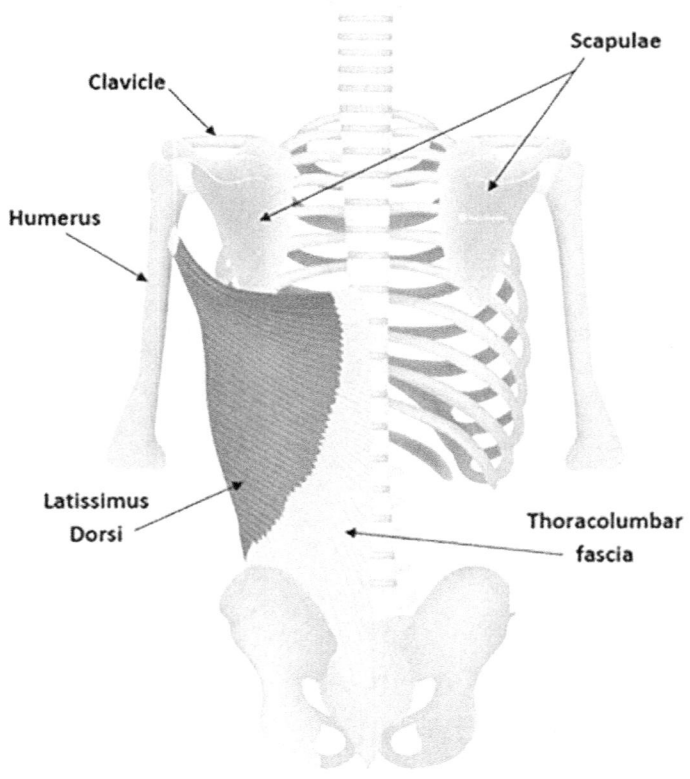

The **thoracolumbar fascia** supports the back muscles and helps them achieve the ability to move the body. It is made up of strong fibers and helps channel forces of movement as the back muscles contract and relax. The nerves to these muscles also cross through this fascia. This fascia goes deep to the spine and is made of three layers. It is essential for contralateral motions like walking. It works with the **latissimus dorsi** (lats) to coil the core of the body.

When the thoracolumbar fascia is supported, it allows all the muscles that connect to it to function better. These muscles include the **gluteus maximus, latissimus dorsi, trapezius, erector spine, quadratus lumborum, psoas, transverse,** and **internal obliques**. It helps bridge the muscles of the back to the muscles of the abdominal wall. This fascia helps to integrate the movements of the upper body with the lower body. Nerves from seven different muscles in the core run through the thoracolumbar fascia.

Latissimus Dorsi: Attaches at the hip and the low back and to the humerus.

It extends, adducts, and rotates inward the humerus. It attaches into the thoracolumbar fascia. It also adducts, extends, and medially rotates the humerus.

See more about the power of the spine muscles and the thoracolumbar fascia in my books *The Power of Your Spine, How Back Strength and Posture Pilots the Entire Body* and *Stroke Recovery What Now? When Physical Therapy Ends, But Your Recovery Continues.*

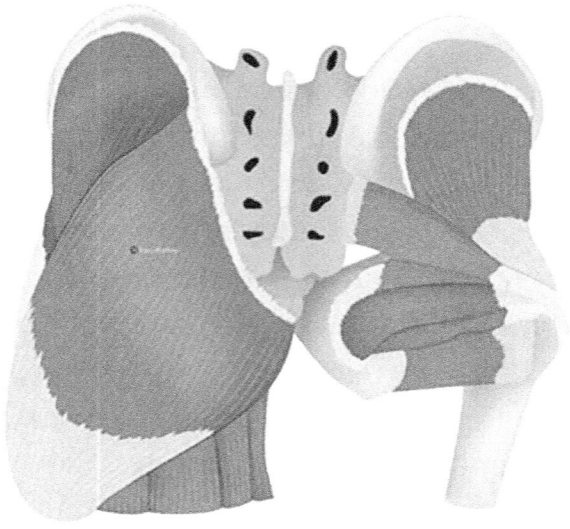

In this illustration, you will see the large glute muscles and the smaller muscles that are underneath. As shown previously in this book with labeled muscles, the large glute muscle extends the femur, which is the backswing of the leg while walking. It also rotates the femur outward. The smaller group of muscles work together to rotate the femur outward.

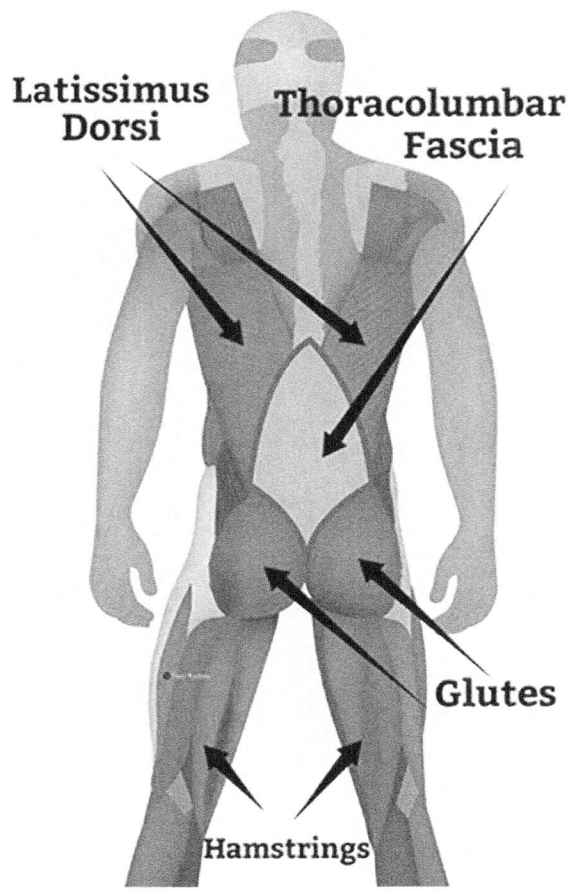

The left **latissimus dorsi** work with the right glutes and vice versa in movements, and walking.

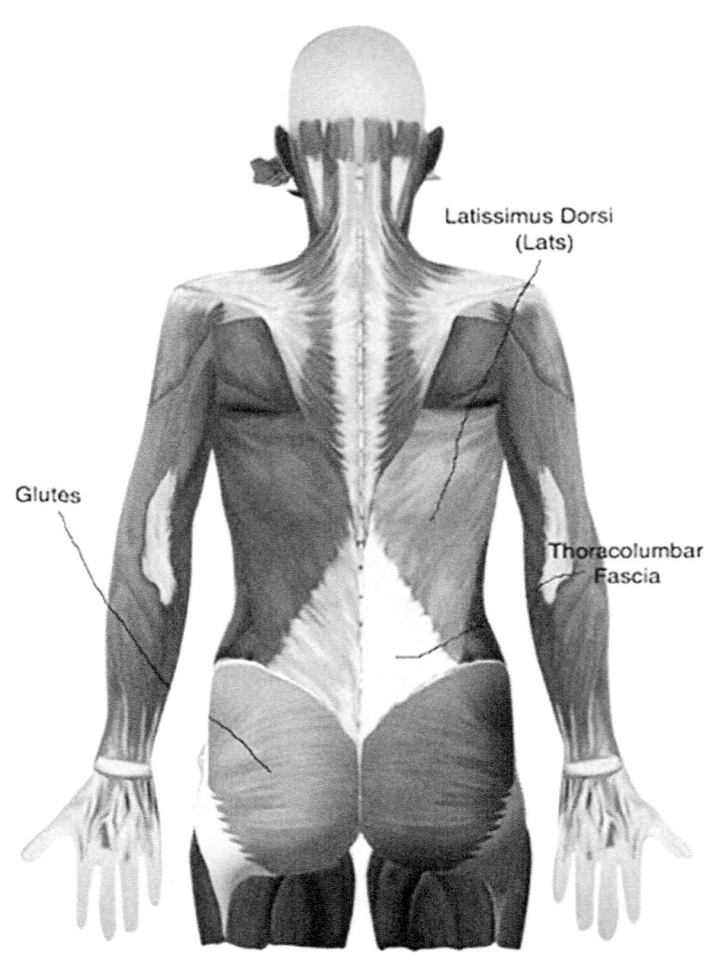

The core must get stronger for the spine to get its natural rotation back for a healthy walking gait. Walking begins at the core.

The Myofascial Lines

I will share a very brief description of the myofascial lines. I also share a few illustrations to give an image to help you better understand movement and how each area of the body can affect the other

The myofascial lines act to transfer the pulling force of one muscle to the other muscles in the body that are connected with each fascial line(s) involved. These myofascial lines are also explained as a line that transmits pulling forces throughout the body. As Thomas Myers teaches in his book, *Anatomy Trains*, this pulling force, also called tension, transfers sequentially from one myofascial unit of the lines to the next. It has been described to be like the dominoes effect. I highly recommend if you are in the fitness industry, a physical therapist, a massage therapist, or other healing professionals, to read the book *Anatomy Trains* and teachings by Thomas Myers.

In stroke recovery, I feel this is great information to help survivors and caregivers to understand more about how, for example, something going on in the shoulder can affect or limit the movements or recovery of the hip and foot, etc. There are many connections through the body like this.

There are many more illustrations to teach these fascial lines. I am just sharing a few of them in this book. This can be complicated, so I am leaving it simple in this book and suggest reading more about it on your own and looking at the many other illustrations available.

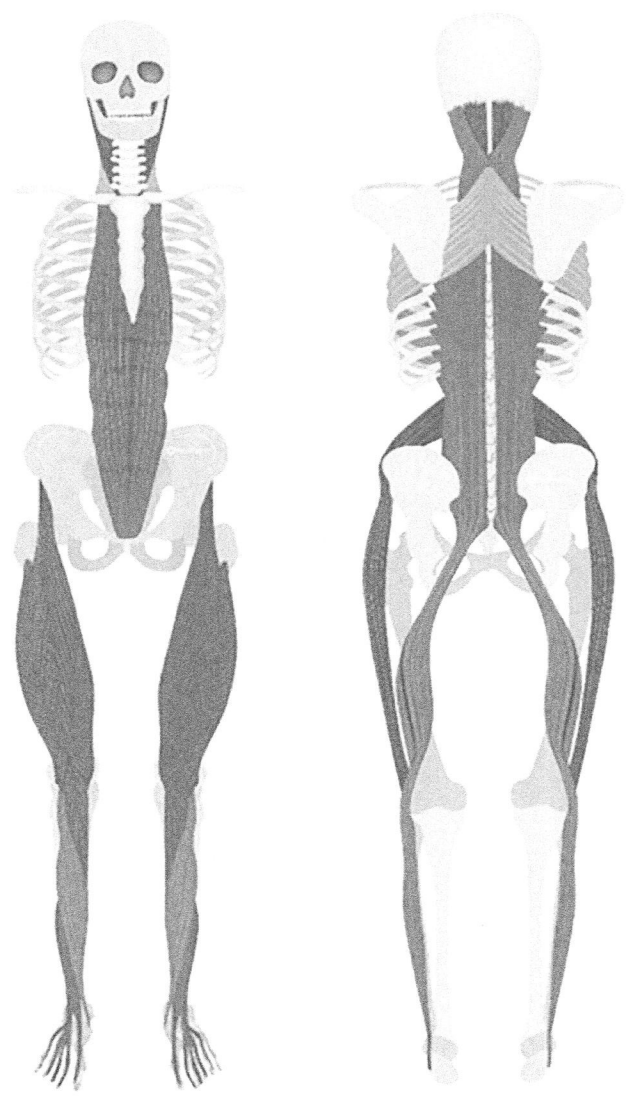

Superficial Front   **Superficial Back**

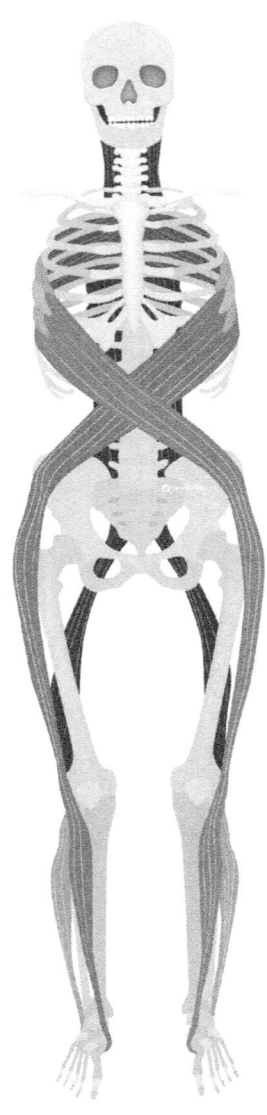

Spiral Line

CHAPTER 7

FASCIA

Fascia is a continuous structure that surrounds and intermingles tissues and structures throughout the body. It varies in density and thickness. Nerves and blood vessels also run through the fascia. When the brain is sending messages for movement, it includes the fascia. Training survivors with knowledge of fascia is important while choosing which exercises are the best for each individual. Fascia is also interconnected with the structures it surrounds. The health and mobility of fascia play a huge role in the body to have healthy movement and to avoid pain and injury. There are ongoing studies on fascia and its mandatory importance for the body to move.

"Fascia contains mechanoreceptors and proprioceptors. In other words, every time we use a muscle, we stretch fascia that is

connected to spindle cells, Ruffini and Paccini corpuscles, and Golgi organs. The normal stretching of fascia thus communicates the force of the muscle contraction and the status of the muscle regarding its tone, movement, rate of change in muscle length, and position of the associated body part to the central nervous system." From Dr. Warren Hammer, the chiropractic profession's leading expert in soft tissues and **fascia,** *"The Fascial System is a Sensory Organ."*

Dr. Hammer went on to say in another article, *"Why We Need to Fix the Mechanoreceptors"* that, *"One of the most relevant discoveries in the world of anatomy over these many years is that muscle spindles, the chief proprioceptive cells affecting our muscles, are not in the muscle, but in the fascia surrounding the muscle and its muscle bundles. A mechanoreceptor is stimulated when it is deformed, but when it is restricted in the fascia that is unable to glide. It is unable to stretch, which is critical for the function of the spindle cell."*

The **thoracolumbar fascia** is an important fascia to understand. It is necessary for walking, running, and mobility. The **thoracolumbar fascia** supports the back muscles and helps them achieve the ability to move the body. It is made up of strong fibers and helps channel forces of movement as the back muscles contract and relax, which is essential for contralateral motions like walking. The nerves to these muscles also cross through this fascia. This fascia goes deep to the spine and is made of three layers. It works with the latissimus dorsi (lats) to coil the core of the body.

When the thoracolumbar fascia is supported, it allows all the muscles that connect to it function better. These muscles include the **gluteus maximus, latissimus dorsi, trapezius, erector spine, quadratus lumborum, psoas, transverse abdominal,** and **internal obliques**. It helps bridge the muscles of the back to the muscles of the abdominal wall. **This fascia helps integrate the movements of the upper body with the lower body**.

CHAPTER EIGHT

THE SCIATIC NERVE

As trainers and therapists, when we hear "sciatic nerve," we instantly think pain. Although the sciatic nerve is said to be the largest single nerve in the body, it is made up of five nerves. It is found on the right and left side of the lower spine by the fourth and fifth lumbar nerves and the first three nerves in the sacral spine. At the largest part of the nerve, it is as big as a male thumb. The five nerves group on the front of the piriformis muscles and become one large nerve, known as the sciatic nerve. **This nerve supplies sensation and strength to the leg and the reflexes of the leg**. It connects the spinal cord with the outside of the thigh, the hamstring muscles, and the muscles of the lower leg and feet. It provides motor and sensory functions to regions of the leg and foot. When the sciatic nerve is impaired, it can lead to muscle weakness and/or numbness and tingling in the leg, ankle, foot, and toes. The sciatic nerve and its nerve branches enable movement and feeling in the thigh, knee, calf, ankle, foot, and toes.

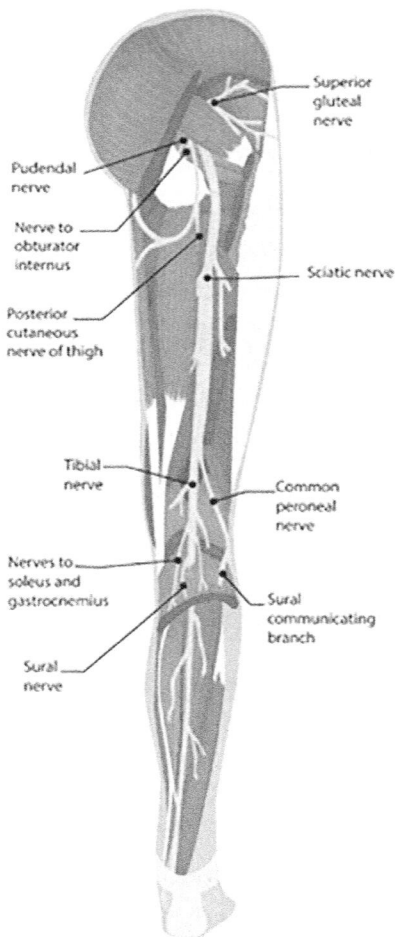

This illustration shows the sciatic nerve and its nerve branches.

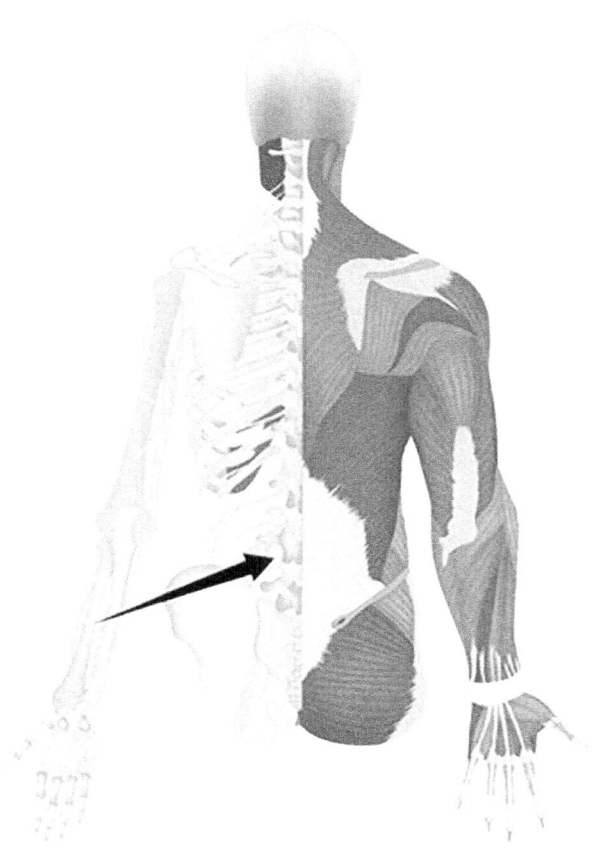

This sciatic nerve exits the spinal cord between the 4th and 5th lumbar vertebrae and travels down both sides of the spine and to/through the **piriformis** muscles. Poor posture and slouching as one sits can affect the low spine and the sciatic nerve. Posture is essential, even while sitting.

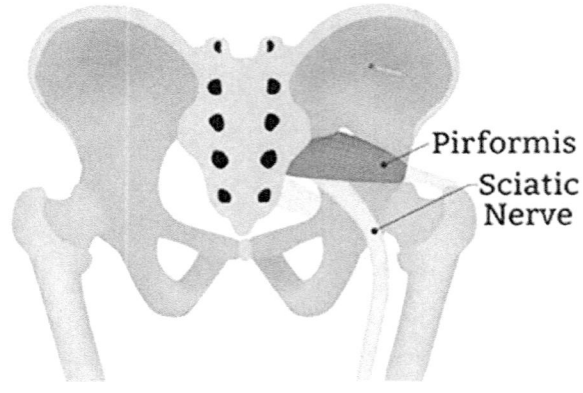

Deltoids
The Shoulder

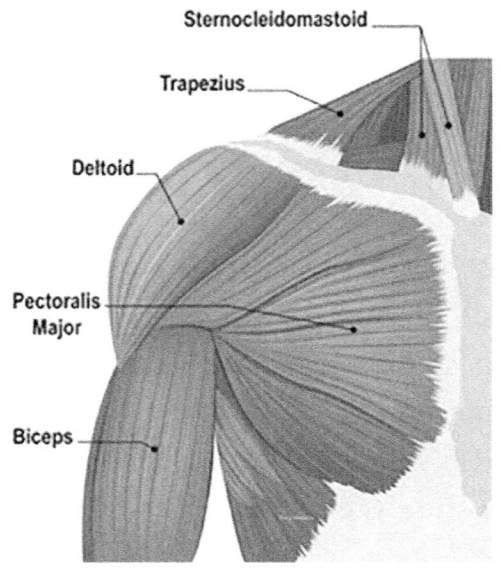

The **Anterior head of the Deltoid** attaches to the clavicle and the humerus.

The clavicle is the collar bone. It flexes, abducts, and rotates the humerus inward.

The **medial head of the Deltoid** attaches to the scapula and the humerus. It abducts the humerus.

The **posterior head of the Deltoid** attaches to the spine of the scapula and the humerus. It extends, abducts, and rotates the humerus outward.

Sternocleidomastoid attaches to the mastoid process, sternum (breastbone), and clavicle (collar bone). It flexes, abducts, and adducts the spine.

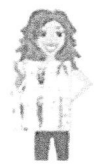 *Reminders and tips.*

Scapula is the Shoulder blade.
Humerus is the upper arm bone.
Clavicle is the collar bone.
Anterior is toward the front.
Medial is in the middle.
Posterior is toward the back.

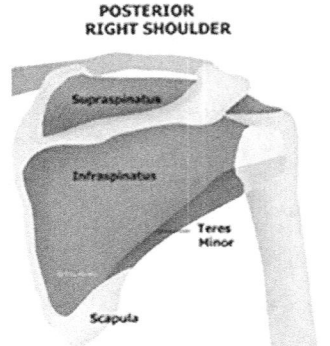
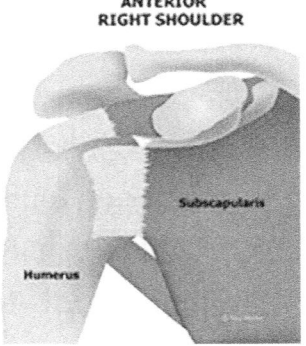

Four muscles make up what is known as the "**rotator cuff**."

These four muscles work together as a team to hold the shoulder girdle properly in place so that the shoulder joint can move freely and safely. These four muscles are the **Supraspinatus**, **Infraspinatus**, **Teres Minor**, and **Subscapularis**. They work as a team, but they also have movements that they perform separately. Using the shoulder joint in exercises and everyday activities in poor posture, will encourage dysfunction and create an injury. It is common for me to hear clients say they have a "rotator cuff injury" and not know which muscle or ligament it is. Many people just assume it is a cuff and do not understand that four muscles are creating the so-called "cuff."

Supraspinatus attaches to the scapula and the humerus. It abducts the humerus.

Infraspinatus attaches to the scapula and the humerus. It extends and rotates the humerus outward.

Teres Minor attaches at the scapula and the humerus. It extends and rotates the humerus outward.

Subscapularis attaches to the scapula and the humerus. It adducts and rotates the humerus inward.

As you can see, all four muscles attach to the scapula and the humerus. However, each of these rotator cuff muscles attaches to different areas of the scapula and different areas of the humerus. To keep it simple, I did not list the exact point of attachment.

The arm and shoulder muscles also play a role in walking. When the arms swing, they bring power in walking. *When the arms are in swinging motion with walking, they encourage the spine to do the natural rotation that performs in the walking motion.* This is another reason it is essential to have good posture, so the shoulders are in the proper position for the arms to swing. In recovery, often, one arm is not cooperating in the movements because of the stroke effect. The arms have a stronger chance of gaining a better recovery when the shoulders are aligned properly for the shoulder's ball and socket joint to move freely. This relies on the body to be in proper posture.

The video at this link https://youtu.be/XguuJXVsb2k is educational and inspiring. It clearly shows how the power of the spine and core is essential for walking. Posture and Core strength are essential. This is not my video. This is the link to the Feldenkrais Move Easy YouTube channel.

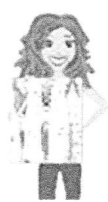

Reminders and tips.

Adduct means bringing a part of the body back to the midline of the body.

Abduction means moving a part of the body further from the midline of the body.

Rotation outward means rotating a part of the body away from the midline of the body.

Rotation inward means rotating a part of the body back toward the midline of the body.

Muscles that attach at the **scapula** and **humerus** must be activated to regain arm movement back. This means performing exercises and movement therapy that move the scapula.

To learn more about the recovery of the arms, see my book, *Stroke Recovery, Regaining Arm Movement.* This book has illustrations of the muscle, nerves, and movements, as well as tips and exercises included.

Keep the shoulder down while sitting, standing, and exercising.

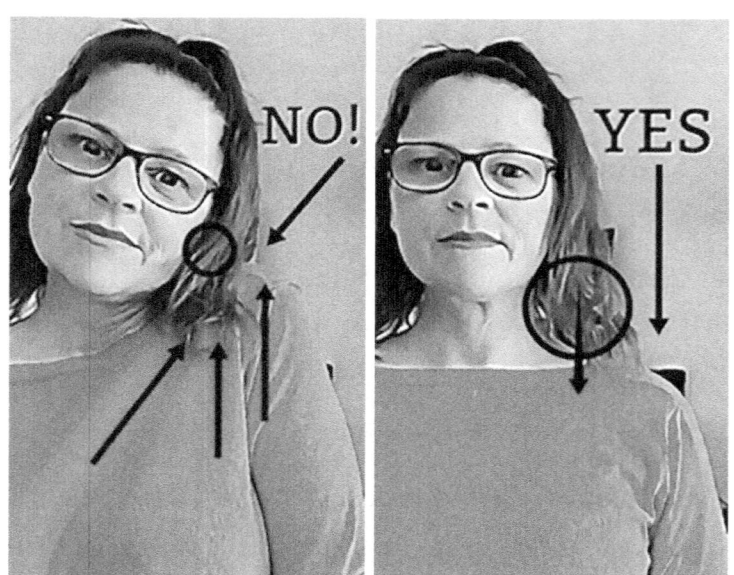

Keep <u>more</u> space between your shoulder and ears, not less.

When you continually have your shoulders raised toward your ears, it puts the shoulder girdle and joint in a poor functioning movement. This will not only cause injuries but put a pull on the fascia that goes through the body and spine.

It also keeps the **trapezius** and some neck muscles in continued flexion. This will cause pain and dysfunction in movements and can lead to more back, hip, and pelvic pain in many people. The stroke survivors that I work with often have a partial or full shoulder dislocation, and if they keep their shoulders down (meaning they stop flexing the muscles that raise the shoulders to the ear), the shoulder can then heal and get back in its proper position. It can also help release hip pain and tightness.

Following the studies on working through the fascia lines, I find the hips and shoulders can inhibit or help each other in individual movements or when they move as a team for body movements. Poor upper body posture will play a role in how your balance, cognitive skills, and walking abilities recover. See the chapter "The Spinal Engine and Working Through the Fascia Lines Theories" in this *book.*

CHAPTER NINE

HAVING A SAFETY BAR
FOR EXERCISE

First, I want to remind you of **the importance of reading the book before just turning to this chapter to do exercises.** The purpose of my books is to help educate professionals, caregivers, and stroke survivors about muscles, movement, exercises, and safety. When you have an understanding of why a specific exercise is being performed and how to do it properly, there is a better chance for further recovery.

Second, **I want it to be clear that having a bar on a wall to exercise with is an essential exercise tool to have in stroke recovery, balance training, and fall prevention.**

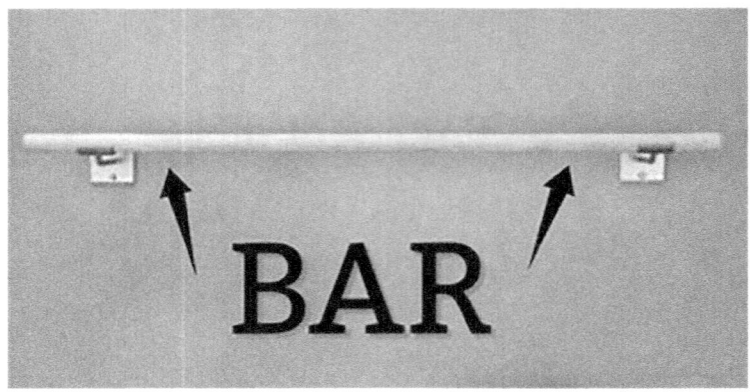

I think the length of the bar should be at least 3 feet up to 6 or 8 feet. This will depend on your space and the ability to have one put in for you. The longer the bar, the farther you can practice walking and taking side steps with it.

One of the reasons it is best to have a secure bar to use compared to countertops and furniture to exercise with is a bar can be grabbed for safety. A countertop and other unstable surfaces keep one at risk to fall, and you are extremely limited to what exercise and advancement you can do. With a bar, you will feel safer and have a sense of control that you do not have without it.

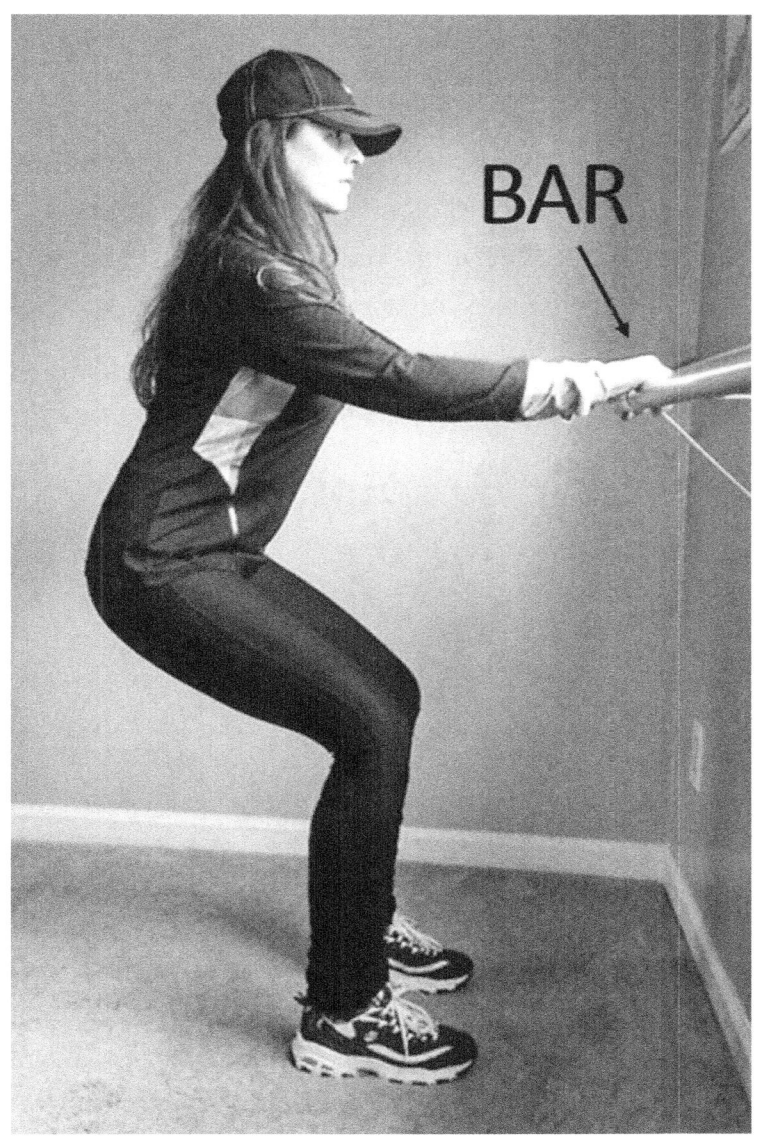

Holing onto the bar and squatting can build the skills and strength to stand and help begin to rebuild a strong core and proper posture. I have mentioned several times in this book, and my other books, that a strong core and proper posture is essential for balance, stabilization, standing, and walking. Keeping a chair under you for safety and as needed as you strengthen is important, as seen in the following picture.

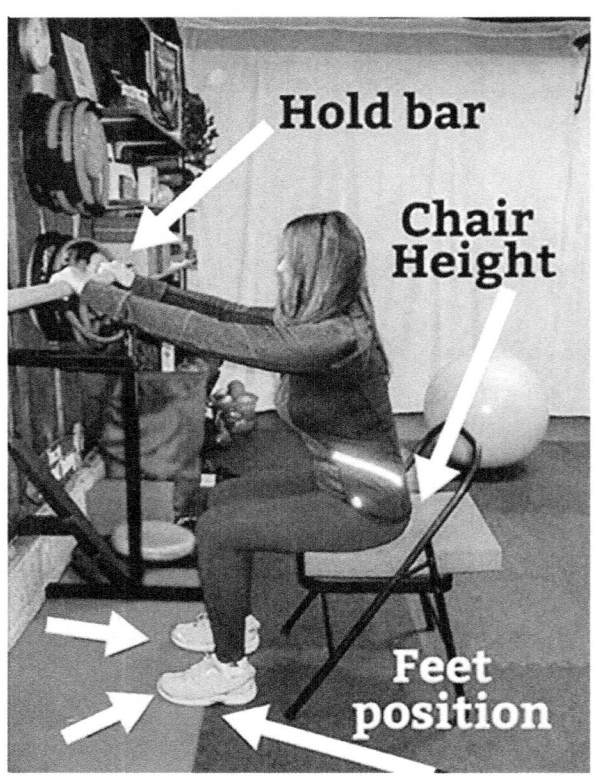

You can put a chair or wheelchair near the bar and practice standing up from seated positions into a tall, proper posture.

Many survivors can only use one arm, as seen in the following picture. In this case, it may take a survivor longer to gain the body strength in the standing and squatting movements because they only have one arm to rely on. Be patient if you can.

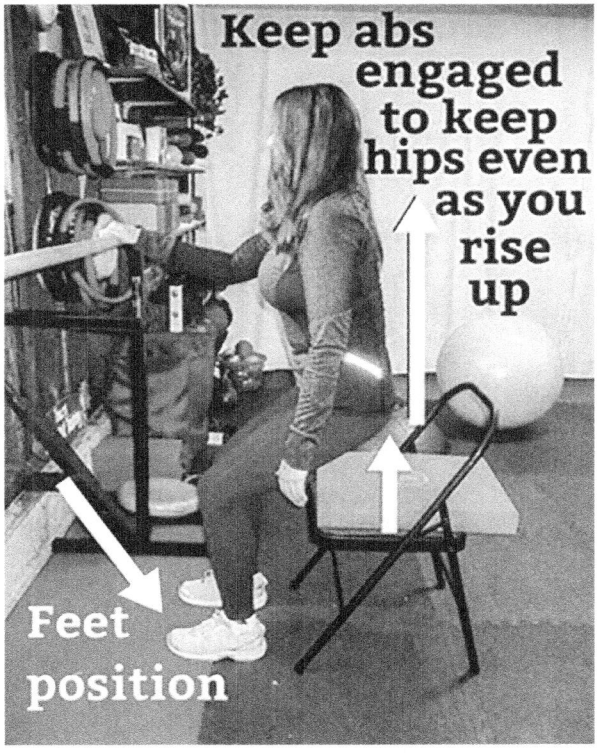

- As you stand up from a chair or a squat position, work on keeping the hips stable by keeping the feet anchored to the ground, and facing forward evenly.

- Keep the abs engaged. This will help *keep the hips from swaying to one side as these movements are performed.*

- Every time you stand up, stand up completely from head to toe.

- Try to keep feet level on the floor. Do not let them roll out to the sides. Keep all toes down, if possible.

- You are building the strength, balance, skills, and pathways to standing up strongly, so walking can become stronger and safer.

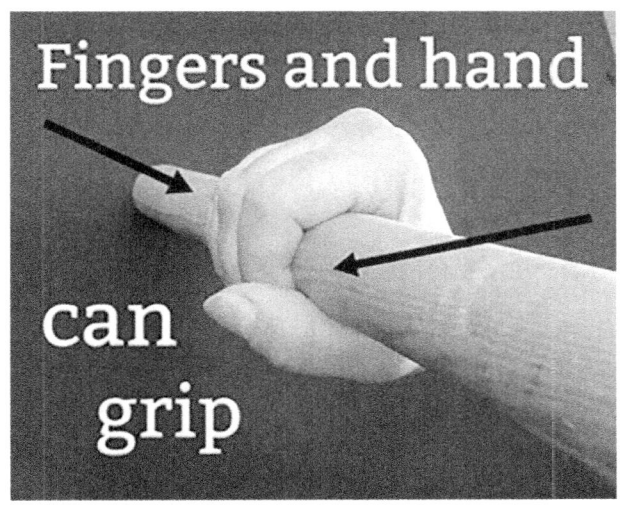

On flat surfaces, such as countertops and unstable furniture, you have nothing to grip onto for safety that will hold your body weight.

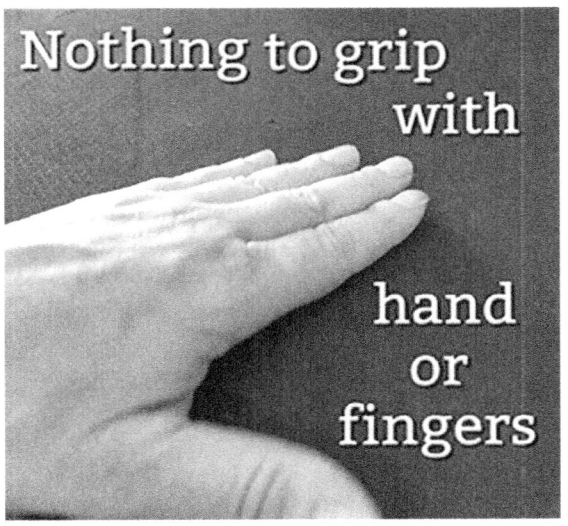

Another plus to using a bar is as your unaffected hand and affected hand (if and when it can) grabs onto the bar, you are using your hands for gripping, grabbing, quick reaction time, which builds stronger arms, wrist, hands and finger strength. The hands and feet can begin to retrain moving and coordinating together with control, rebuilding pathways to arms, hands, and fingers, and much more.

Safety First!

With the hand challenges, many survivors face practicing, gripping, and releasing the affected hand from the bar is good for hands that grip too much and for the hands that will not grip at all.

As you review the different exercises in this book, please take note that not all survivors are at the same place in recovery. There will be exercises that one survivor can do that another survivor cannot do. All survivors must begin at their own starting point and advance at their own pace.

When you see the exercises standing on balance pads, BOSU® balls and discs, know to

ALWAYS begin standing on the ground first using the bar.

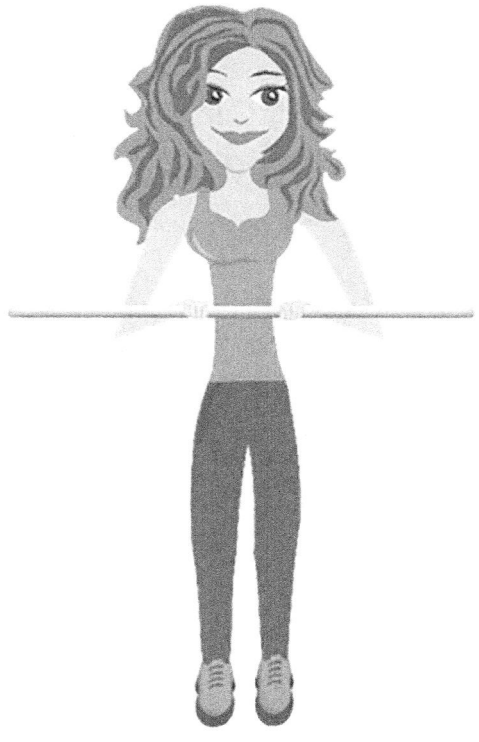

When you are needing to practice standing up from a chair or a wheelchair, use the bar. Each time you stand up, try to engage your abs and stand completely up.

Many times, when people are struggling with balance, stabilization, and walking, they do not complete their stand up and try to take steps with the body in poor posture. This makes it harder and risk for falls. **<u>BUT</u>**, if you are having trouble and feel UNSAFE, **<u>USE THE BAR</u>** until you can feel safe and ALWAYS have someone with you to work with. If possible, find a trainer or therapist to keep you **<u>SAFE</u>**.

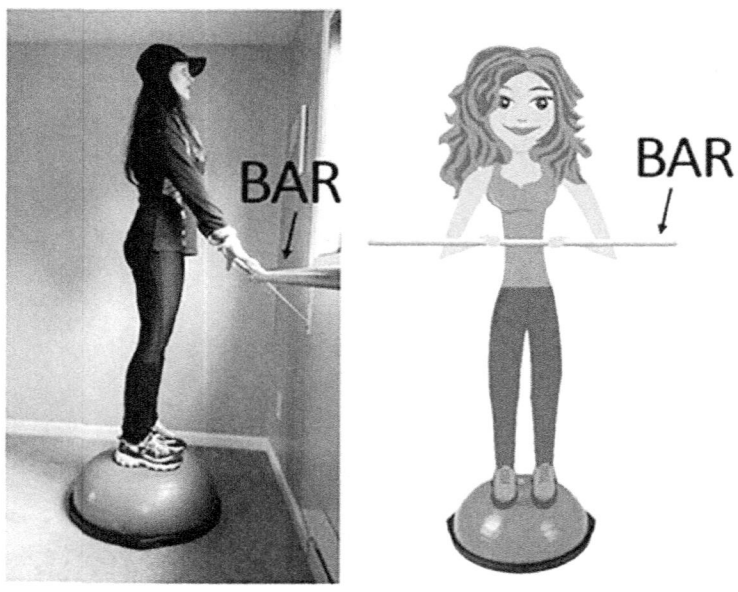

Safety First!

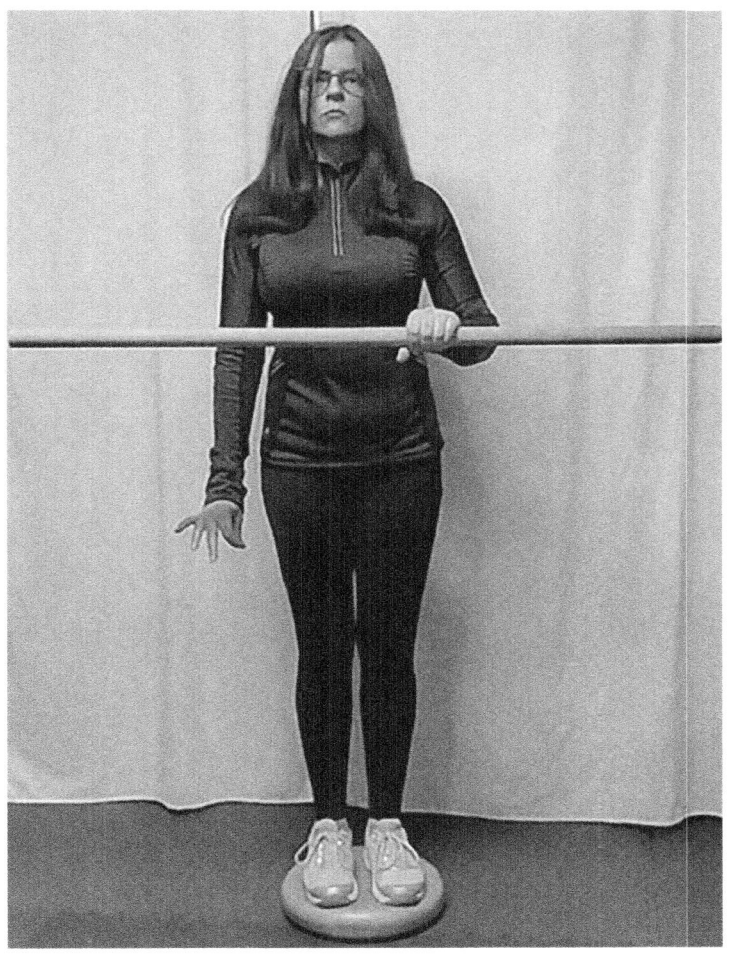

Hold onto a bar for safety.

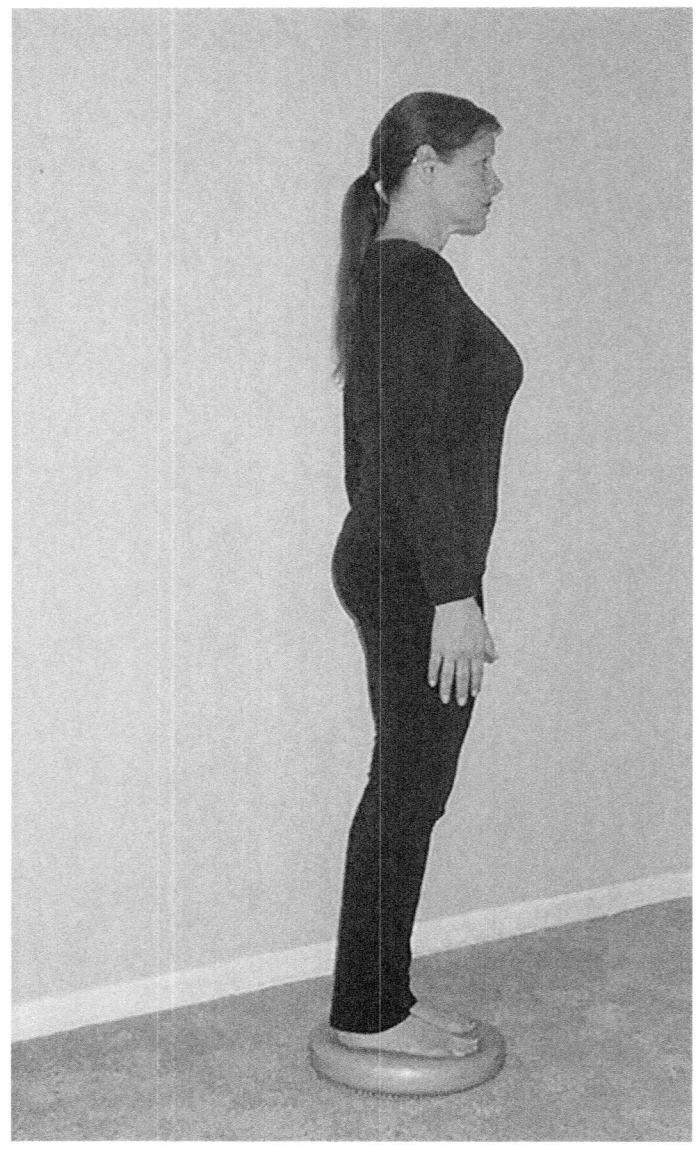

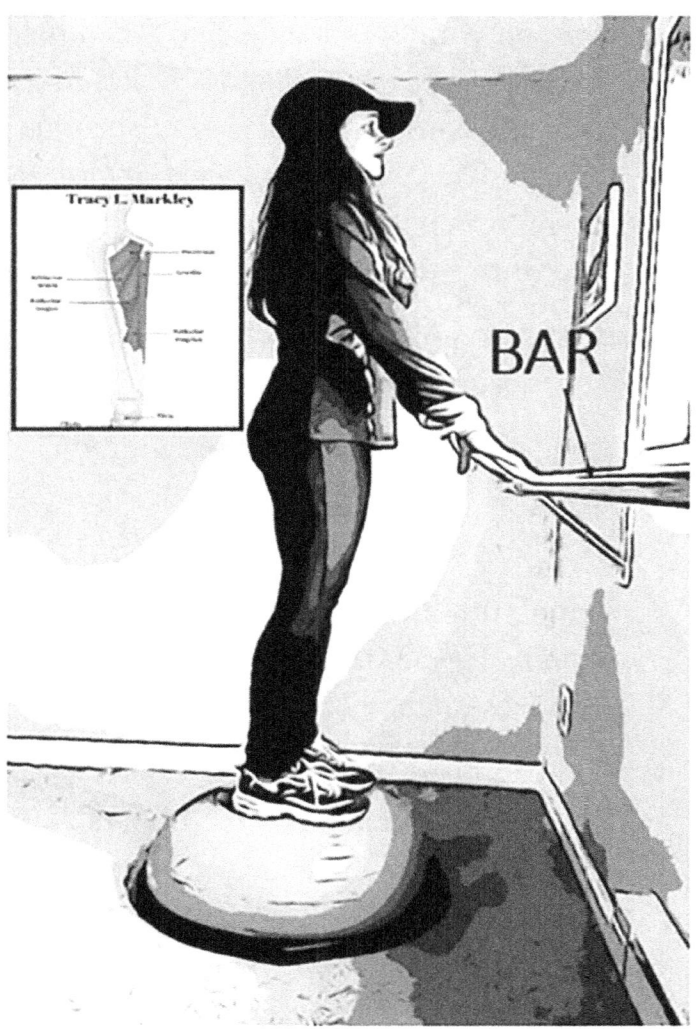

Standing on a BOSU® ball also exercises the muscles in Illustration in resistance training. Remember, these muscles help to hold the femur bone (upper thigh bone) upright and stable for standing and walking.

- Hold on with both hands, and when ready, you may rotate both hands by holding on with only one hand for a few seconds or longer. This will all depend on each person's personal case and ability at the time of exercising.

- Be sure to hold onto a secure object such as a bar secured to a wall.

- Stand in a proper posture with the abs engaged.

- If you are doing arm and hand exercises as shared in my book *Stroke Recovery, Gaining Arm Movement*, if possible, do the exercises on the non-affected hand first.

- The exercises shared in this book can be done sitting, standing on the floor, standing on BOSU® ball, balance disc, balance pad, kneeling on a BOSU® ball, sitting on a ball, or sitting in a chair. **Ensure your safety first**. Then when ready and safe, you can try the more advanced ways.

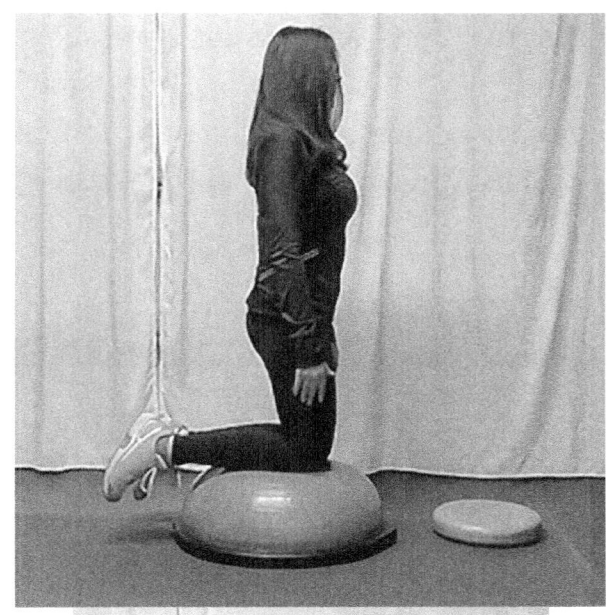

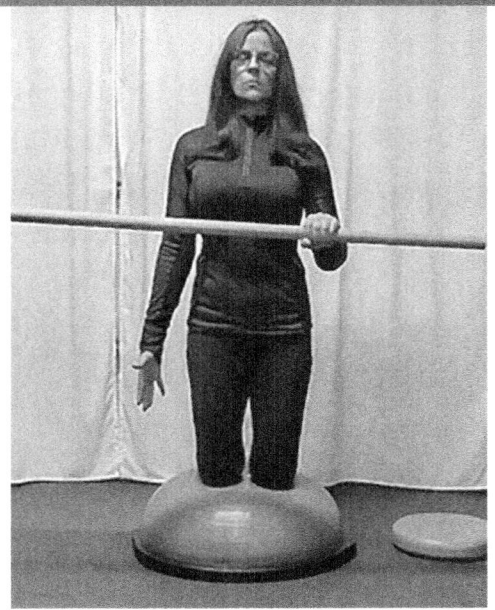

- As the core and postural muscles gain strength to hold your body upright in the proper posture, balance, stabilization, and arm movements can gain more recovery.

- Kneel in a proper posture with the abs engaged.

- Sit with proper posture with abs engaged.

- When you engage your abs, DO NOT squeeze your butt muscles.

Currently, most of you have already been through therapy, or you are still receiving therapy. Either way, remember this book is filled with knowledge and exercises to possibly assist you in recovery. As I mentioned earlier in this book, I am not a physical therapist. I am a fitness trainer who often works with clients who have finished their physical therapy and do not know what else they can do or how much further their recovery can go. **The stroke survivor's recovery does not end when physical therapy ends.**

You may only be able to do some of the exercises here as well as some of what your therapist has shown you. Do the exercises that you can do and can do safely.

- Begin with core and postural exercises.

- Standing on a balance pad, disc, BOSU® ball, or kneeling on BOSU® ball is a great way to warm up the core and postural muscles. This also strengthens these muscles and stimulates the central nervous system. It also helps train the body to multitask again and helps to rebuild special awareness and quick reaction time. This builds balance and stability. These are excellent warm-up and exercises to do for fall prevention.

- If you are unable to use balance props, begin standing on the floor until you are safe and/or advance.

- Move the shoulders and the shoulder blades.

- Get the muscles and nerves deep in the spine activated by standing on one of the balance tools or sitting on a ball (when ready).

- Move the shoulders/arm through the different movements (that are on the page on shoulder joint movements) the best that you can.

- The shoulder joint movement exercise can also be done, sitting, or standing with or without the balance tools. Always be in a proper posture when exercising. **Safety First!**

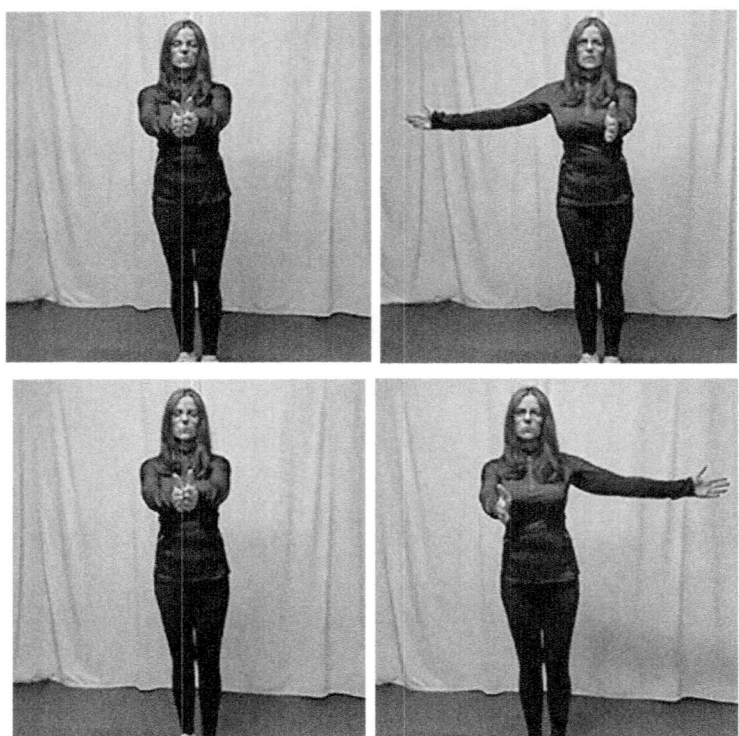

With the exercise above, really focus on where the hands and arms are in space. Try to control the height of both arms, making the goal to keep the hands meeting in the center of your body and staying at the same height as you gently and slowly move your arm to the side and bring it back slowly with control.

Using bands can be a great source with the correct posture and positing. In the following pictures, I am demonstrating my exercises using the Anchor Point Training® Band. These bands also come with a neuro handle. This handle helps stimulate nerves while doing the exercise. I have found they work fabulously with stroke survivors.

The next exercises help with spinal posture/proprioception and balance as well as purposely being aware of where the arms are in space. This can be done standing, sitting in a chair, wheelchair, or on a ball. Have your feet on the floor. The disc under my feet is more advanced. As with any exercise you try, try the beginning steps first; then advance when ready. **Safety First!**

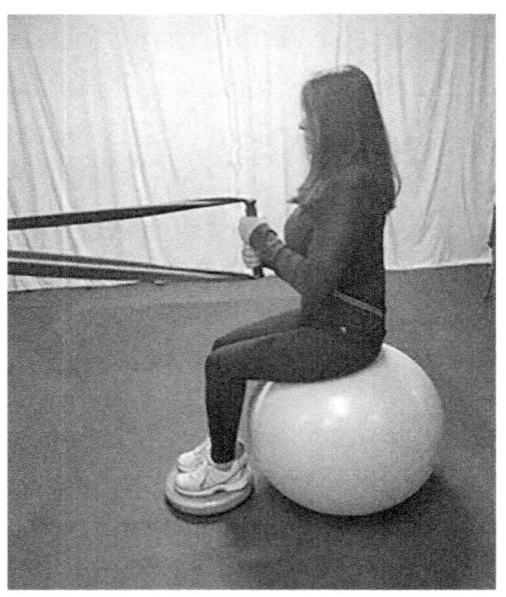

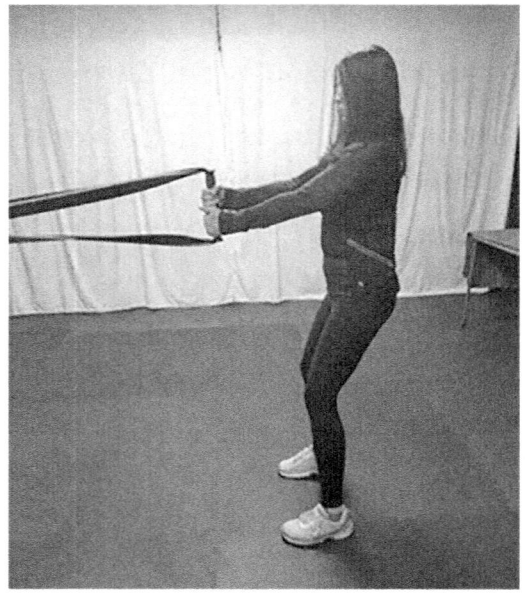

In the picture with me sitting on the ball (in the correct form), I also have my feet on a balance disc as I perform the exercise. This is more advanced. Straighten the arms with control and pull the band back towards your chest. I am also using the neuro handle from Anchor Point Training®. The brain is working extra hard as I am keeping my feet in good positing and maintaining proper posture as I do the exercise. This will also be a good time if you have someone with you to gently move their fingertips along the spine in the area where the nerves exit the spinal cord. See more about this and other arm exercises in my book *Stroke Recovery, Regaining Arm Movement.*

- Do the exercise that you can that you have learned in this book and the exercises you learned from your therapist if you feel that they are still helping you. Some of the exercises may be the same.

- If you are not too exhausted, repeat some things.

- Listen and feel what your body is telling you.

- There will be days when you will get exhausted quickly, and other days you can keep going. Respect your energy level each day.

- See my videos at my YouTube channel at *Tracy L. Markley Fitness* https://www.youtube.com/channel/UCQbpnj-LoB0R3nm7V2p_MLA

When I train my clients in private, I can give directions for their personal needs at that moment in their recovery and where their progress is gaining.

This book contains tips and some of the exercises I do with clients.

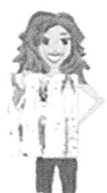

Reminders and tips.

Warming up the spine, upper back, and arms through exercises can also help you before you work on your standing exercises. I suggest just doing a few of the exercises, if possible. This way, you warm up and get the shoulder blades moving and do not overwork the arms, so they end up being too tired to assist with standing and walking exercises.

Remember to pace yourself and honor your journey and recovery path.

CHAPTER TEN

EXERCISES AND TIPS

H ere are some important exercises that I have found to be essential to regaining balance, strength, and stability for safe movement. Depending on the client, I may have them start by sitting on a Swiss ball, standing on the balance disc, or I may have them start by standing on the BOSU® ball. In all cases, especially in the beginning, I have the client hold on to a ballet barre or the squat rack bar, even though I am in the fitness studio. If you are trying these at home, be sure to have a safe item to hold onto.

In each standing exercise:

- Engage your abs. Imagine you are zipping up a zipper to put on a snug girdle.

- Be aware of your body's location in space from head to toe.

- Be aware of feet placement. Feel them evenly anchored wherever you are standing. Try to keep feet evenly placed; do not let them roll out to the sides.

- Stand up tall, stack the shoulders over the hips, and imagine you are lengthening your spine to the sky.

- Imagine your body weight is lifting as your feet maintain the sense of being anchored in the ground.

- For safety, when needed, hold onto a bar or secure object, which allows you to maintain a good posture.

- Hold on enough to be safe, but do not become so stiff that you do not feel the balancing challenge of the disc or BOSU® ball.

- If you are sitting on the stability (Swiss) ball, anchored as described above, keep the knees over the ankles and sit up tall with your shoulders over your hips.

- Follow the instructions and tips listed with each of the following exercises.

- **Safety First!**

Sitting on a chair and/or sitting on a stability (Swiss) ball

- Begin this exercise sitting on a chair or a bench of the appropriate height.

- Directions listed here apply to sitting on chair, bench, or ball.

- **Safety First!**

- When balance is stronger, and it is safe for you, it can be done on the stability ball.

- Be sure the ball is firm.

- Be sure the ball or chair is the right height for you. Your hips should be level with your knees. **Do not sit on a mushy ball or on a ball where your hips are below your knees**.

- Sit on the ball or chair so that your lower legs are as close to the ball as they can be **without touching** it.

- Keep your knees directly over your ankles. This means your shin bone will be in a straight line from the ankle to the knee. Think of table legs coming directly out of the table joint, which allows the table leg to be positioned straight up and down.

- Do not let your knees fall in or fall out, and do not squeeze your legs together.

- Anchor your feet into the floor.

- Engage your pelvic floor (if possible) without squeezing your butt muscles (glutes).

- Engage your abs like you are putting on a snug girdle.

- Stack your shoulders over the hips.

In the beginning, a survivor may feel that there are too many things to remember. That is okay; it is normal. Keep focusing from head to toe. This will help the body and brain regain better communication consciously, which will help rebuild the communication subconsciously as you strengthen the muscles in your spine and core.

A survivor's stroke-affected leg may fall out to the side, and they may not be able to hold a ball between their legs without assistance from their hand or a professional. I like to have the survivor sit in a chair near a wall. I then place a ball between the wall and the affected leg. Then they can use another ball between the knees to do the exercise the best they can.

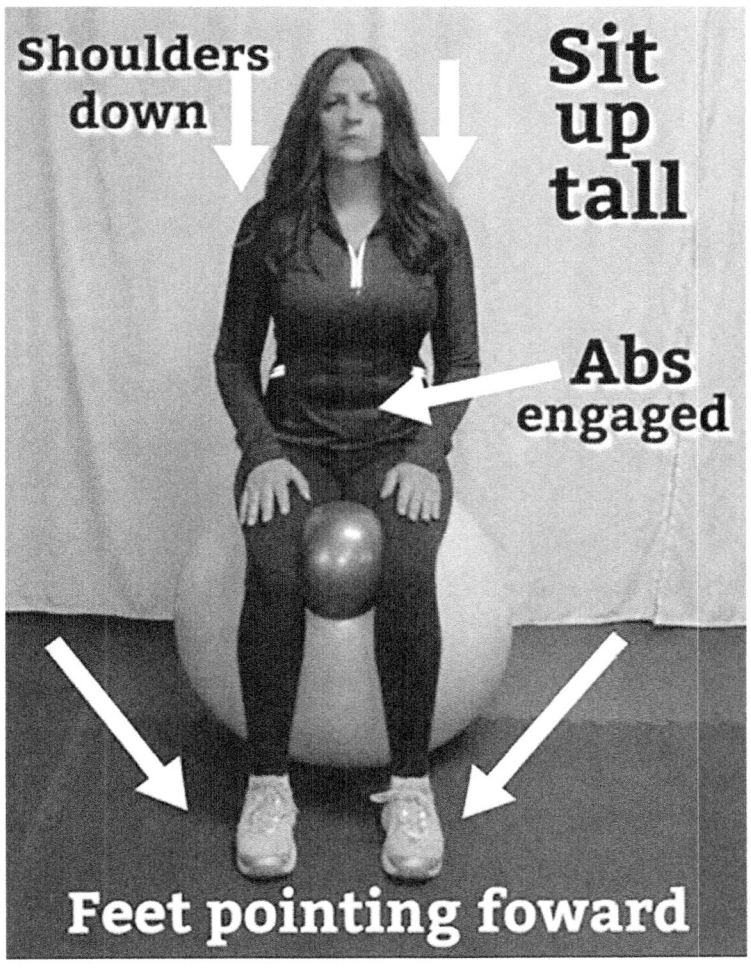

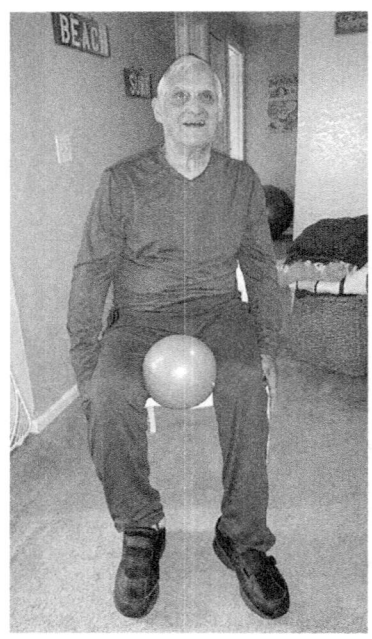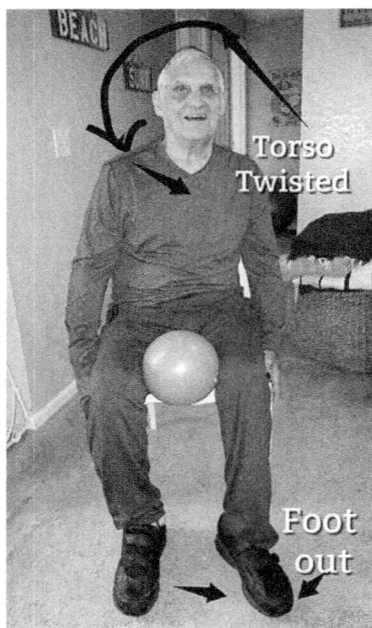

In the previous two pictures, you can see that he is sitting with his upper body in a twist, and the left foot is turned out. Your body may want to do this automatically but work on keeping the proper positions with the feet and posture as in the previous picture with me illustrating the proper setup.

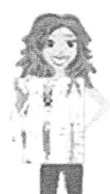

Reminders and tips.

- Remember when a foot turns out, it turns the leg out up to the hip and pelvic. This leaves the hips, pelvic, and spine in an uneven position. You want to build the body evenly, not unevenly.

- Remember, studies show that when the body is in proper posture, all the systems work better.

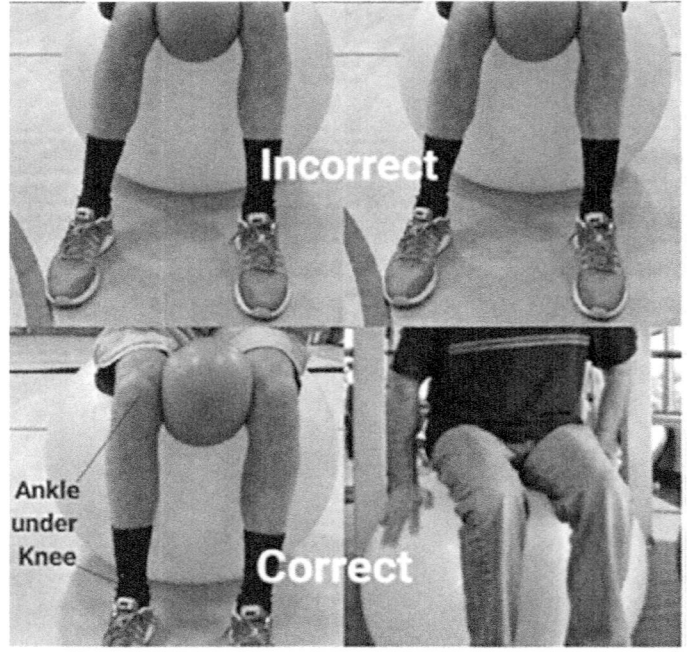

Do these exercises in a chair before you advance to a ball.

Sitting on a chair or a Stability (Swiss) Ball - Adductor/Abductor Exercise

Use a Bender® ball or a small soft Pilates ball and gently squeeze between the knees/inner thighs. This can be done with your feet flat on the floor and tiptoes.

- Set up in proper posture and positioning on the ball or chair.

- Place the ball between your knees or inner thighs, wherever it feels comfortable for you.

- Recheck your position and posture and feel as if you are putting on that girdle and lengthen the spine up tall with the abs engaged.

- Gently, but firmly squeeze the ball between your knees (inner thighs) with control, then release with control. Repeat this movement for 10 to 20 reps. Be sure to use the same speed throughout the exercise. (Try NOT to squeeze the ball and then quickly "snap" the release.) Work yourself up to three sets of 20 reps. (This number changes and varies per person). When I am working with a client, we communicate and determine together the number that works for them based on the strength and ability of the client.

- **DO NOT** squeeze the butt (glutes) while performing this exercise. For most people, this takes focus.

- As with any exercises, if your back, hip, or knee joints hurt while doing this exercise, first recheck your form, and if that does not fix it, **STOP** the exercise!

- It is never a good idea to hurt one area of the body to strengthen another. Proper exercises that works for the whole body, while avoiding injuries, is essential.

- As you advance with this exercise, and it is safe for you to do, you may place a balance pad or balance disc under your feet as you sit in the chair or the ball. This will bring more of a challenge in balance, stability, spatial awareness, proprioception, and neutrally.

Standing on the Balance
Pad and Balance Disc

If you are using a balance disc, the disc mustn't be too flimsy. I have found that the CanDo® brand, 35cm/13 inches, is a good one to use. I have found mine on Amazon.

- Engage your abs. Imagine you are zipping up a zipper to put on a snug girdle before even stepping onto the balance disc. Re-engage your abs once you are standing on the balance disc.

- Be aware of the body's location in space from head to toe.

- Be aware of feet placement. Feel them evenly anchored where you are standing. Try to keep your feet evenly placed; do not let them roll out to the sides.

- Stand up tall, stack your shoulders up over your hips, and imagine you are reaching the top of your head to the sky.

- Imagine your body weight is lifting as your feet maintain the sense of being anchored to the ground.

- Hold onto a bar or secure object so you can maintain a good posture, but do not hold the body so stiff that you do not feel the balancing challenge of the disc.

- Depending on each survivor's balance strength or challenges, one must **always** begin at their own level.

Beginning with a balance pad before the disc is also suggested and often needed.

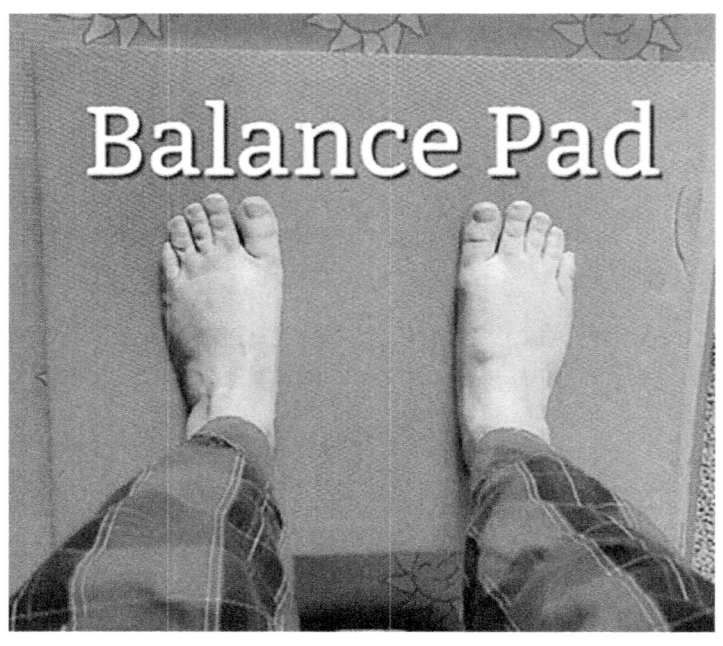

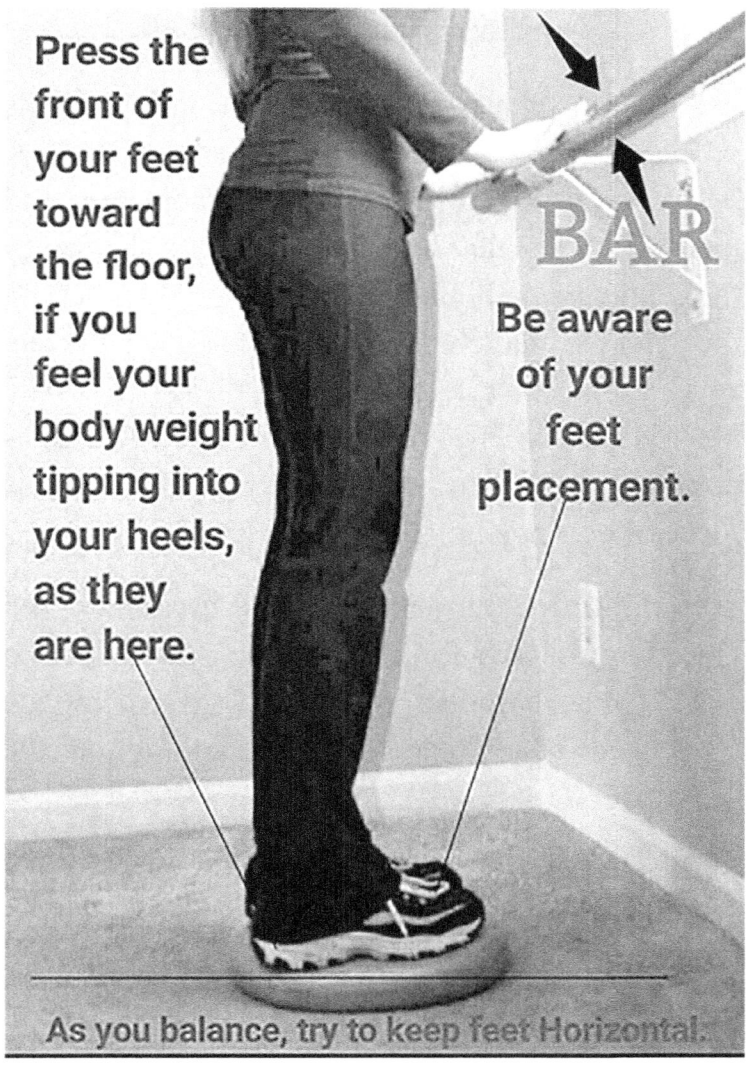

Press the front of your feet toward the floor, if you feel your body weight tipping into your heels, as they are here.

BAR

Be aware of your feet placement.

As you balance, try to keep feet Horizontal.

The above directions are the same that apply while standing on the ground, a disc, a pad, or the BOSU ball®.

Standing on the BOSU® Ball

You must have the BOSU® ball inflated to its proper firmness. Usually, if you turn the BOSU® ball over so that the platform is facing up and measure the distance from the floor to the top of the platform, it should be about 9 to 10 inches off the ground. I have noticed that BOSU® balls can vary a bit in size. A flatter ball DOES NOT MEAN IT'S A BETTER CHALLENGE. That is not how it works; it is not the science behind this piece of equipment.

- Engage your abs. Imagine you are zipping up a zipper to put on a snug girdle before even stepping up from the floor. Re-engage your abs once you are standing on the BOSU® ball.

- Be aware of your body's location in space from head to toe.

- Be aware of feet placement. Feel them evenly anchored to where you are standing. Try to keep your feet evenly placed and do not let them roll out to the sides.

- Stand up tall, stack your shoulders up over your hips and imagine you are reaching the top of your head to the sky.

- Imagine that your body weight is lifting as your feet maintain the sense of being anchored.

- Hold onto a bar or secure object so that you can maintain good posture, but do not hold the body so stiff that you do not feel the balancing challenge of the BOSU® ball.

- Depending on your individual balance strength or challenges, you must **always** begin at your own level.

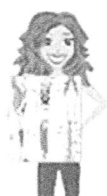 ***Reminders and tips.***

Practice standing on the ground with the bar first, until you are strong enough and stable enough to try it on an unstable surface.

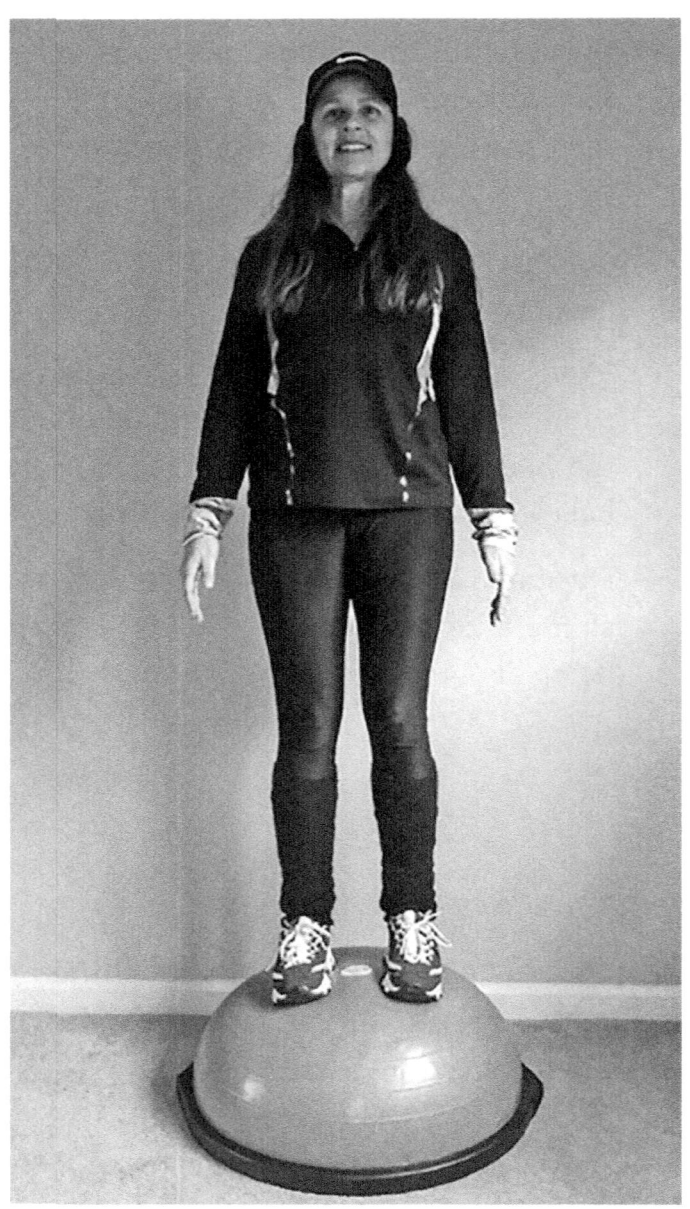

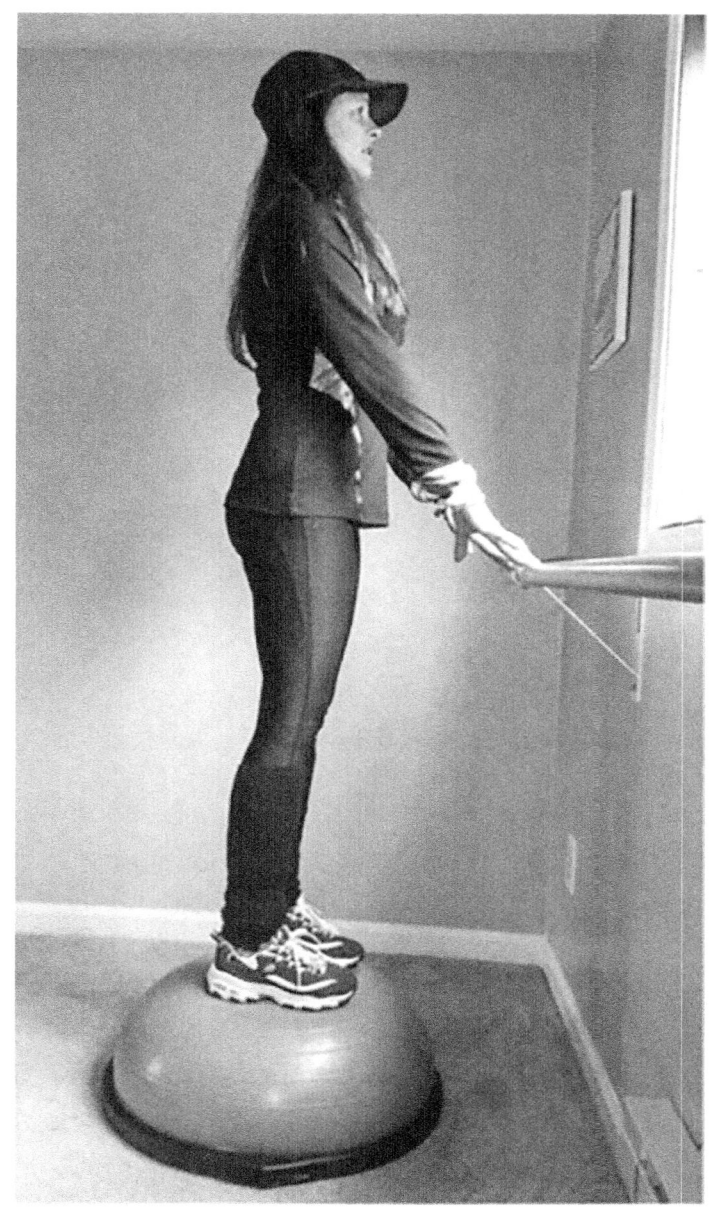

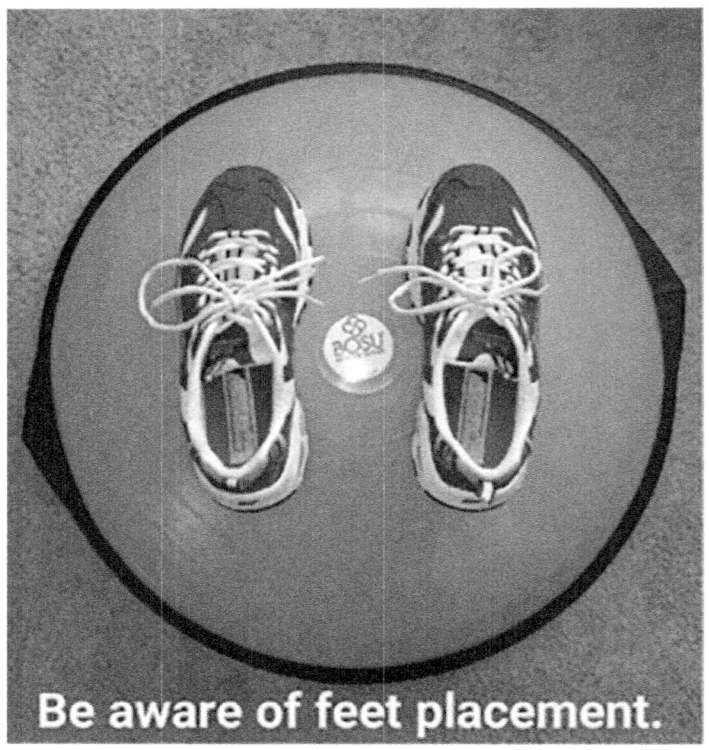

Be aware of feet placement.

- To begin, take a step out, then bring the feet together, then step to the side again.

- **Safety first!**

- When you are more advanced, you can put an exercise band on the bar to add more strengthening and balance. I like to use the Anchorpoint Training Bands, as seen in the next pictures.

- I particularly like using the Anchorpoint Training Bands with the special neuro handles.
- Find out more about these bands on my website. www.tracyspersonaltraining.com

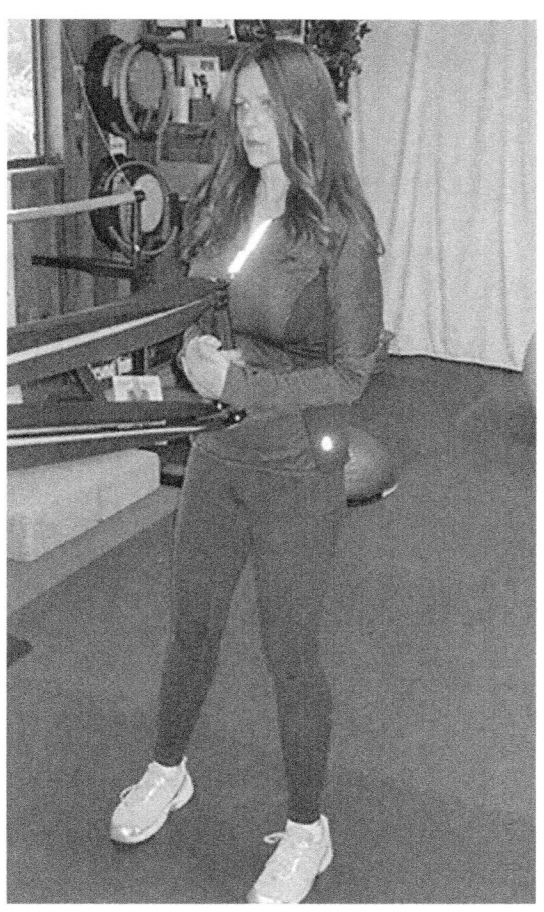

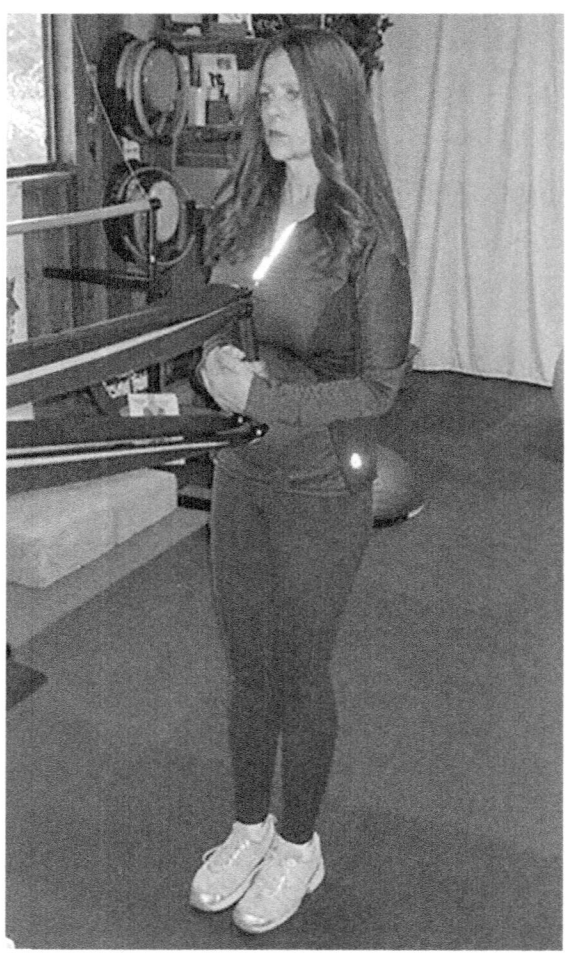

Taking side steps while holding onto a band as I am doing in the pictures works balance, stabilization, posture, core, spatial awareness, and proprioception as well as practicing the steps in movement.

Taking Steps to the Side

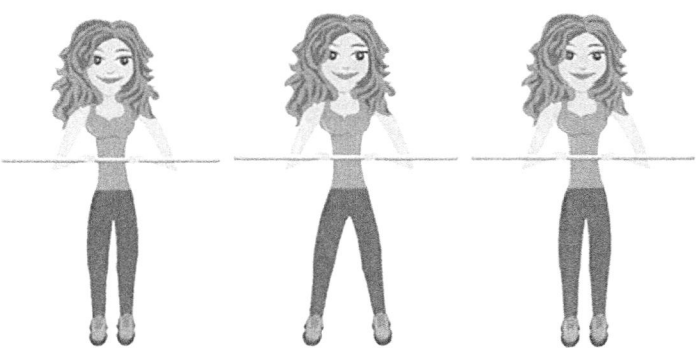

- Hold the bar for balance and safety.
- Try not to tense the arms, shoulders, and neck while holding onto the bar.
- Stand tall.
- Abs engaged.
- Relax shoulders. Keep the shoulders down away from your ears.
- Try to keep the foot that turns out directed forward, like in the illustrations.
- Start with feet together, then step one foot out, then bring the other foot to it.

- Take steps sideways in both directions the whole length of your bar.

- Try to keep the feet pointing forward through the movements.

- This exercise will help fix foot drop, drag, and hyperextended knee if you are very aware and focused on each step.

- Try not to let the foot drag in your steps.

- Lift each foot consciously off the ground while taking each step.

- Do this along the bar as many steps as you can take (depending on the length of your bar), then go back the other direction.

- Stay upright in proper balance.

- Try not to drag either foot.

- Stay aware of what both feet are doing in each step. This is spatial awareness. You are also trying to regain spatial awareness of where your feet are in space. **This is a part of fall prevention training**.

- Try not to let your hands pull you in the side steps. Holding on to the bar is intended to keep you safe and balanced so that you can work on your feet' steps and posture.

- Taking side steps while being focused on each placement does a few things.

  1. This makes one focus on where the feet are in movement.

  2. While taking steps, purposely placing the foot in the proper position (not turned out) keeps the hips and the muscles above the foot in their correct positions, which strengthens them in the correct positions for keeping the foot in control unconsciously again.

  3. If you are able, try not to let the foot drag, by purposely lifting the foot off the ground for each step.

  4. This is one form of "knowing where your feet are in space," also known as spatial awareness and part of proprioception.

If you are unstable and unsure of your balance and coordination, have someone always with you while you do your walking and stepping exercises. Holding onto the bar and taking side steps back and forth across the length of the bar helps the hip and leg abductor and adductor muscles as well as practicing and regaining the connection to the spatial awareness of where your feet are in space.

Practicing Walking

If you are unable to use a treadmill to practice your walking on, use the bar.

When practicing walking, **ALWAYS** use the bar if you are unstable, and you have balance and stabilization challenges still. Stand sideways close to the bar and hold on with your stronger side's hand. Always check your posture, stand tall, and practice your walking in good form. Remember to go your own pace and the stroke-affected pace you need to be at to be safe.

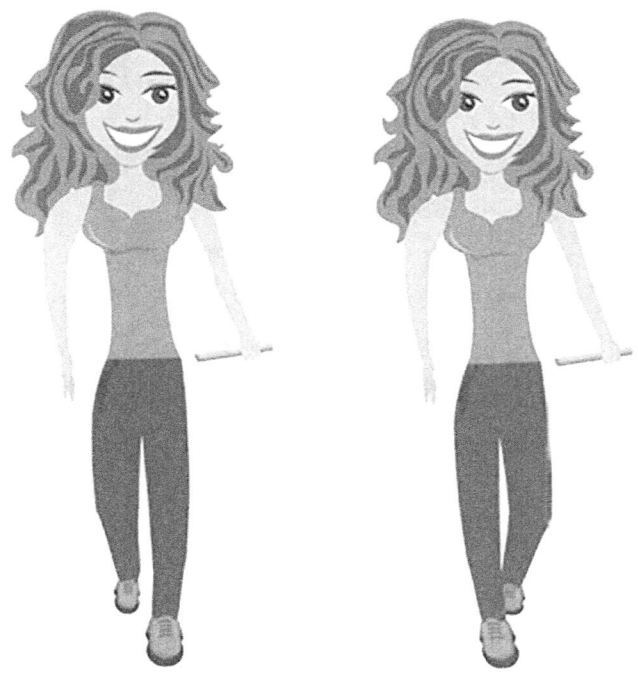

If you can, try to keep the foot from dragging and/or turning out while you take your steps, by purposely lifting the foot off the ground for each step.

Walking Backward and Backward Movements

Walking backward might seem silly, but it is good for you physically and mentally. We take steps backward often in our daily activities. Walking backward enhances the sense of body awareness. It increases body coordination and movement of the body in space. Research has shown walking backward improves forward walking skills. It is said to sharpen your thinking skills, enhance cognitive control, and put the senses into overdrive. This movement also puts less strain on and requires less range of motion from the knee joints.

Everyone needs to have awareness as to where the "body is in space." Athletes need to practice and train with focused awareness on where their body is in space for function, speed, and agility. They gain better balance, speed, and quicker reaction time, which are incredibly important skills for sports, especially fast-moving sports. Stroke survivors need to regain these skills for everyday life movements and regain quick reactions. Some examples: if they drive; moving quickly to the brake pedal when needed; moving their foot quickly to avoid tripping and falling or avoiding dropping an object on the floor.

I have heard trainers suggest having a client walk backward on a treadmill to help increase awareness and foot placement, but I am **NOT comfortable** with that. I feel walking backward on a treadmill belt **IS UNSAFE**. I suggest having a survivor do it on the floor in front of a mirror so they can see and feel the foot placements. If you do not like looking in the mirror, watch your feet and walking gait in the mirror.

REMEMBER TO USE A BAR.

Practice walking forward every day. Be sure you are not alone or have a professional with you if you are unstable. **BE safe!**

Only practice walking backward if you can safely do so.

Walk alongside the **bar** to hold onto it.

If you do not have control of placing each foot exactly where you want it when you step, walking backward will not be safe to do. **Safety First!**

After doing the previous exercises for some time, the ability to walk backward may feel safe again.

If you are unstable and unsure of your balance and coordination, have someone always with you while you do your walking and stepping exercises.

If you are using a walker, DO NOT DO THE WALKING BACKWARDS EXERCISE.

Stepping on and off the BOSU® ball

- USE A BAR FOR SAFETY IF NEEDED!

- Engage your core as explained in Exercise 1 or for the balance disc before even stepping onto the dome of the BOSU® ball.

- Spend a few minutes standing and balancing.

- When you are ready to step up and down, remind yourself to stay focused and mindful of each foot's placement as you step up and step down.

- Come to a complete balance once both feet are on the dome. Stand up tall, stacking your shoulders over your hips.

- When you feel balanced, stay focused, and then step back to the floor.

- Once you come to a complete balance on the floor, stand up tall, stacking your shoulders over your hips. Then step back onto the dome.

- If possible, begin by stepping up with the right foot and stepping down with the right foot. Do this five times; then switch to stepping up with the left foot and stepping down with the left foot.

- Work yourself up to 10 on each side.

- If you personally have a foot drag, a drop challenge, or another physical challenge or weakness, making this difficult to do, *KEEP PRACTICING.* It may get easier with time. But **safety first! The more you are repetitive with a movement, the better chance the brain has of making**

the new pathways needed for such a movement.

- When stepping off to the floor, focus on clearing the dome. The goal is not to let your foot drag down the dome or hit the plastic platform. If you have extra physical challenges, this movement will come with time. *KEEP PRACTICING.*

- When finished with stepping up and down, go back to just standing and balancing. You will find you can balance better now. If the first few times you do not experience this, it will come with time. *KEEP PRACTICING.*

This is an especially important exercise to help you regain balance and rebuild a safe and strong walking gait. It helps to rebuild an awareness of the location of your feet in space during your movement.

We take small steps stepping backwards many times each day:

- When we open a door towards us.
- When we approach a chair to sit down.

- Doing laundry.
- Stepping down a ladder or step.
- Backing away from the bathroom or kitchen sink.
- Using your feet to push yourself in a chair away from a table before you
  Stand.
- And more.....

If you are having a hard time with the exercise of walking backwards, begin with the exercise of stepping up and down on the BOSU® ball first, and/or include it in your workout program before you work on walking backward.

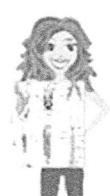 ***Reminders and tips.***

Remember, the brain sends a message to the deep core muscles to stabilize the body before movement.

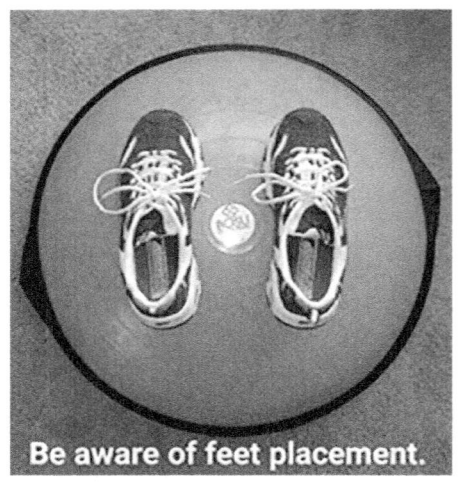

Be aware of feet placement.

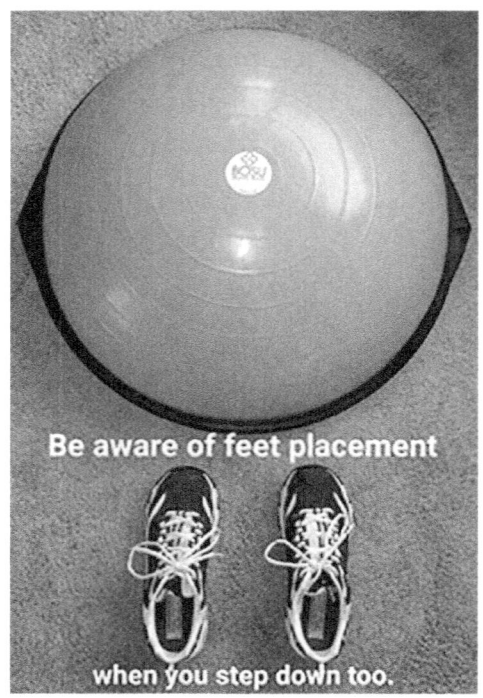

Be aware of feet placement when you step down too.

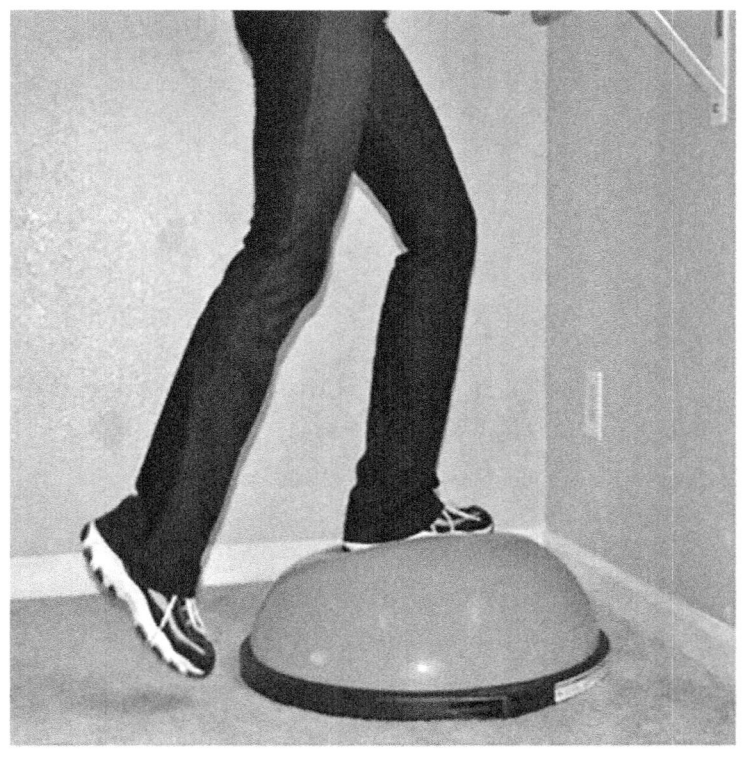

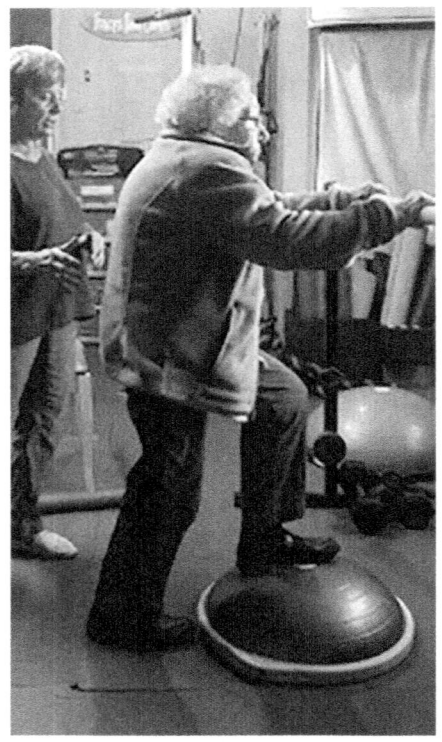

If you are unable to step on the standard BOSU® ball, use a child-size BOSU® ball if you are able. The client in this photo was only 4 feet 11.

You can also use a box or a step that is safe to use as an exercise prop for stepping up and down, as shown in the next pictures.

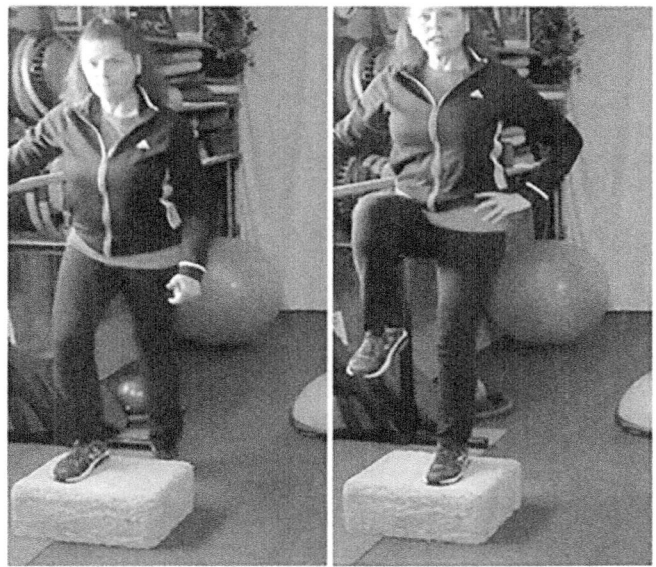

Two different exercises are being shown in these pictures.

The *1ˢᵗ Picture is demonstrating basic stepping up and down.*

The *2nd picture is more advanced.* This is stepping up and lifting the leg high, then stepping back down.

The first exercise is beginning for re-learning stepping up on steps. The use of the BOSU® ball is more advanced.

- In all the exercises for stepping up and down, use the bar for safety.

- Engage your abs and stand in good posture.

- Step completely onto whatever you are stepping on. Do not let part of your feet hang off the prop you are using.

- If you are using the BOSU® ball, step completely onto the center of the ball. See feet positions while standing on BOSU® ball in this book.

- Step both feet completely on to the step, balance pad, or BOSU® ball.

- Once you have both feet on your stepping prop, stand tall and be in good posture before you step back down off the prop.

- As you step off, focus on clearing the prop that you are using.

- Once both feet are on the ground, stand tall and get in a good posture, before stepping back up again.

- This may take time and lots of practice. Remember that you are also re-training spatial awareness of where your feet are in space as you move back to step down as well as when you step up.

- Only do this exercise and any exercise if you are safe.
- Remember **Safety First!**
- In time this can help you be safer taking stairs.

Squats Holding on to a Bar

This exercise can be done standing on the floor or standing on a balance pad or the BOSU® ball.

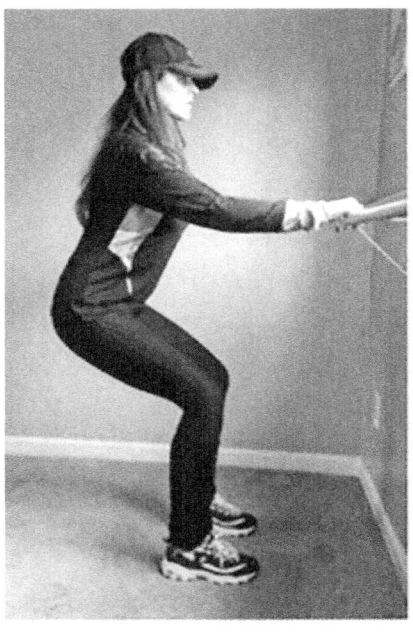

Be sure you can do this on the ground <u>before</u> attempting it on a BOSU® ball.

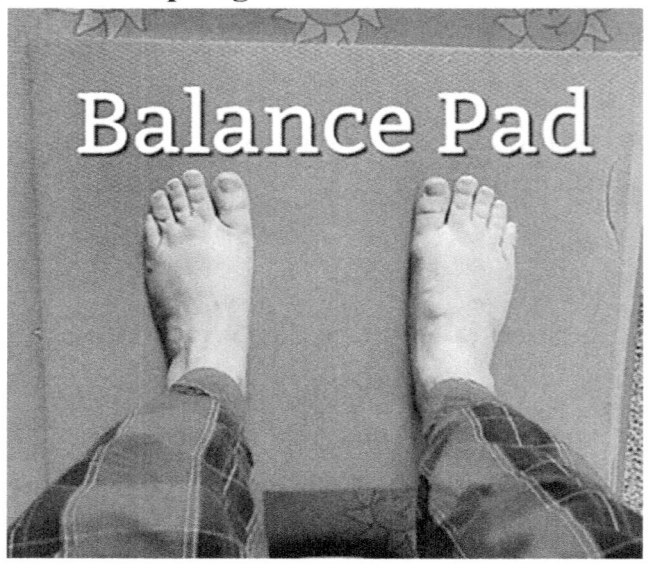

When using the balance pad, you can be barefoot or wearing shoes. Proper foot placement is the same as with the disc and BOSU® ball

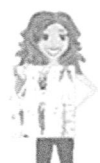

Reminders and tips.

It is a **wise** idea to practice standing on the ground first.

When you are ready, practice on the balance pad.

Then when ready advance to using the balance disc and BOSU® ball.

Safety First!

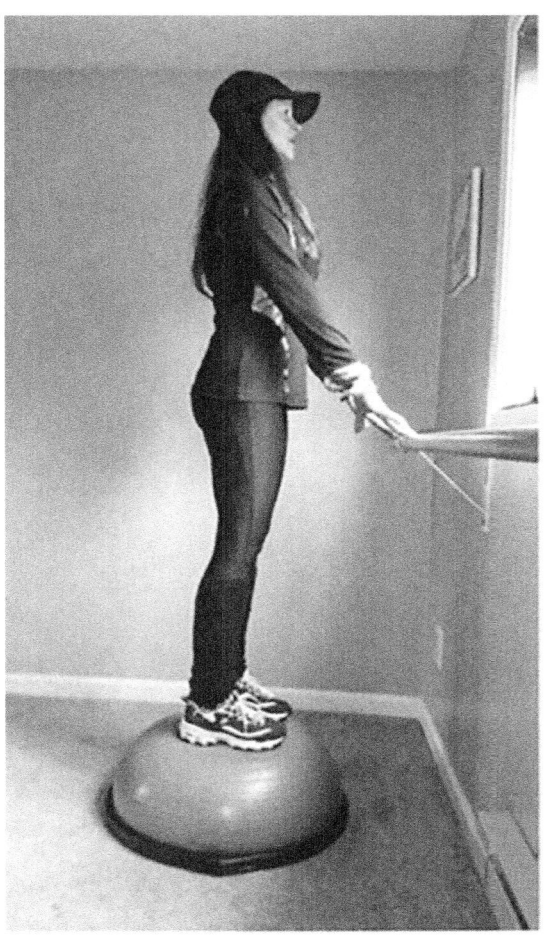

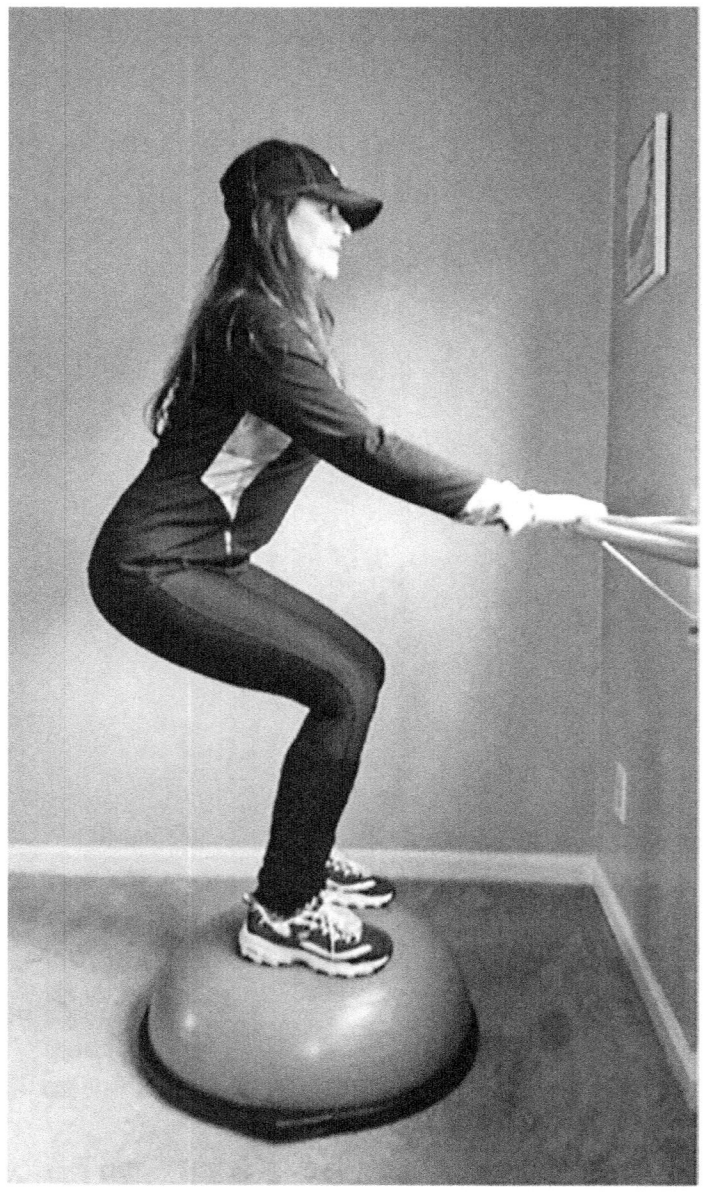

This exercise is more advanced, and some survivors can do this, and others may not. Remember to work at your own pace and ability.

- Begin by doing this exercise with your feet on the floor first. Be sure you can hold the proper alignment safely before you begin performing this on the dome of the BOSU® ball. You can also do this standing on a balance pad. When you are stronger, you can do squats with the BOSU® ball. **Safety First!**
- While facing the bar, evenly hold on to the bar with your hands, so that your body is centered between your hands.
- Engage your core and focus. Hold the body in good form from head to toe, including the shoulders.
- Sit back as if you are going to sit in a chair, then raise yourself back up.
- Try to use your legs and glutes to do the movement. Do not allow the arms to do all the work.
- Do not drop the hips below the knees.

- If this bothers your knees, check your form. If it still bothers your knees, do not do the exercise.
- If you are doing this standing on the floor, pull yourself up to a good posture between each squat.
- If you are doing this on the BOSU® ball, pull yourself up to good posture and balance yourself straight up and down in good form between each squat.
- Maintain control and focus throughout each movement.
- In each squat, make sure both feet are parallel so that your hips and pelvis are moving evenly through both sides throughout each rep.
- If you are using the BOSU® ball, do about 8-10 squats; then spend a couple of minutes balancing on the BOSU® ball. When you are stronger, work up to three sets of 10 squats, balancing in between.
- Work your way up to the squatting. Depending on each individual's ability, a survivor may not feel safe to do the squats in the first few weeks or even months.
- **Safety First!**

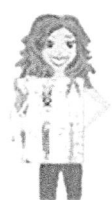

Reminders and tips.

Extra Tip: Often, if a survivor puts a bean bag on their head, it helps with posture. This helps connect the sensation to where the head is in space and helps lengthen the upper torso into a better posture.

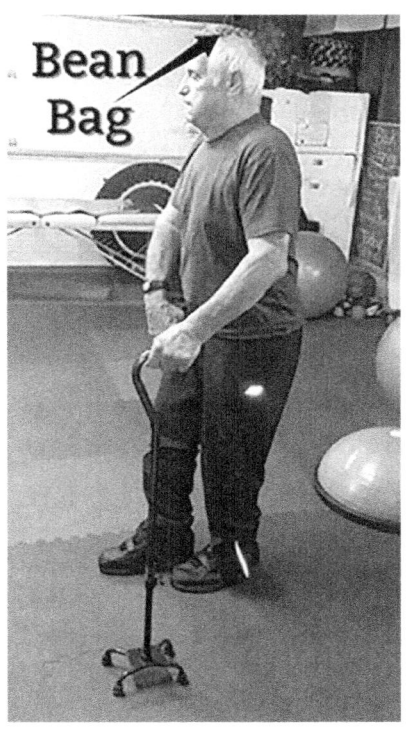

Battling Ropes

Battling ropes, also called battle ropes, are a great tool for stroke survivors and those with balance and neurological challenges. They work well for neurorehabilitation for stroke, brain injuries, cardiac rehab patients and are excellent for age-related disease. Battle ropes have a low risk of injury and are non-impact weight resistance. There is a 2-vector force direction created while using the battle ropes. This means that one direction of force is pulling away from the person while a downward force from the pull of gravity from the weight of the ropes. This causes multiple contractions of different muscle groups at the same time. As this is taking place, the ropes challenge the dynamic balance and stabilization while using them. They are being used more and more for rehabilitation and corrective exercises. They help with asymmetrical stabilization issues. Depending on the recovery stage in a stroke survivor, one may only use one rope at a time or two ropes at a time. There are different wave patterns to use with the ropes that create velocity and challenges the core muscles in different patterns.

Individuals can use ropes in wheelchairs and walkers. They can be seated in their wheelchairs or on a chair that is an appropriate height for their height and hip level. They can be used sitting on a ball, standing on the floor, and standing and sitting on the BOSU® ball, squatting, lunging, kneeling, and more. I took a Battling Rope Coach Certification course with NESTA to better my knowledge using the ropes with clients. There is much more to battling ropes then I am mentioning in this book.

There are hundreds of exercises that can be done with them. The ropes come in different lengths, diameters, and weights.

Here are a few basic tips. Understand the purpose of the different hand grips. Maintain proper posture. Have the shoulder girdles set in proper alignment.

A survivor may be able to use both ropes at once, or they may use a single rope. It will depend on the individual challenges they are working through. The way the hands grip the battle ropes make a difference. If an individual has an arm that will not work well with the ropes yet, use a single rope with the double hand grip. If possible, perform the exercises in one position; then rotate the hands, so the other hand is on top and perform the exercises again. The stronger arm, of course, will be in control, but the other arm will follow in movement and participate in the exercise as well, but with guidance from the other hand. I suggest performing making waves with the battle ropes and the tsunamis. These can be done standing or kneeling on the ground, sitting in a chair, wheelchair, roller walker, Swiss ball, standing, and sitting on the BOSU® ball.

Different Hand Grips May Be Used While Using Battle Ropes.

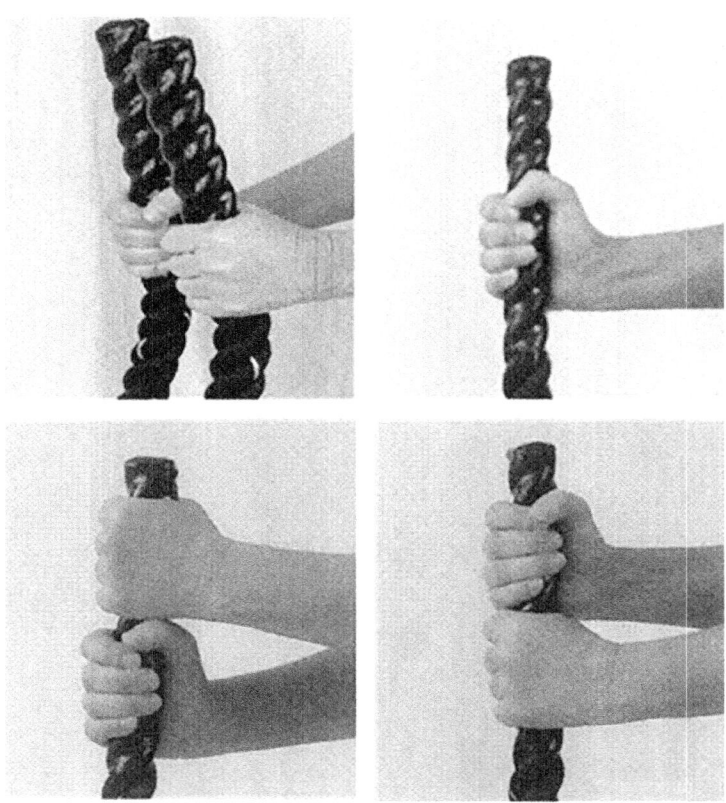

In this hand grip, as the client performs Waves or the Tsunamis exercises with the battle ropes, the push muscles are being worked

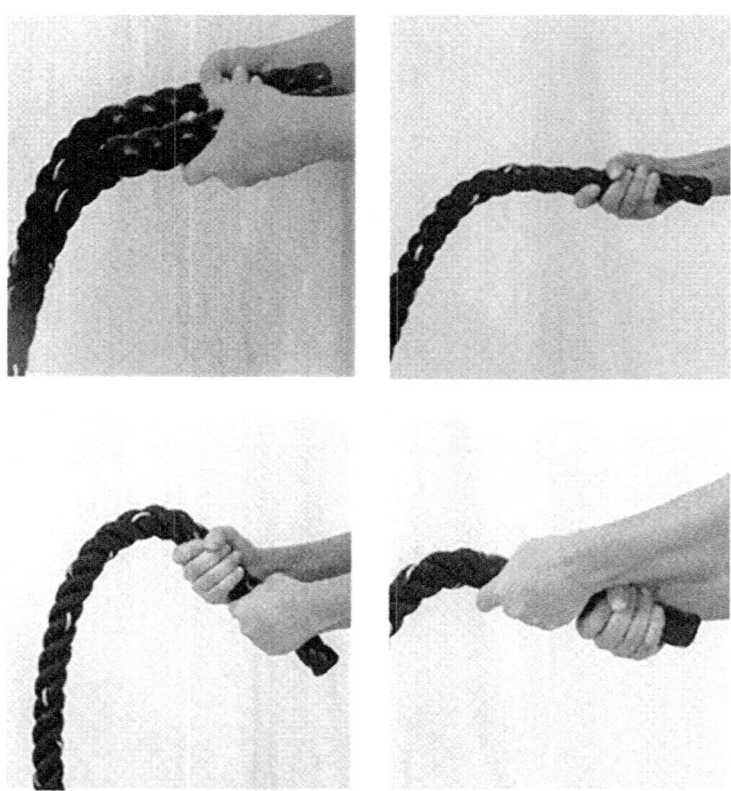

In this hand grip, as the client performs Waves or the Tsunamis exercises with the battle ropes, the pull muscles are being worked

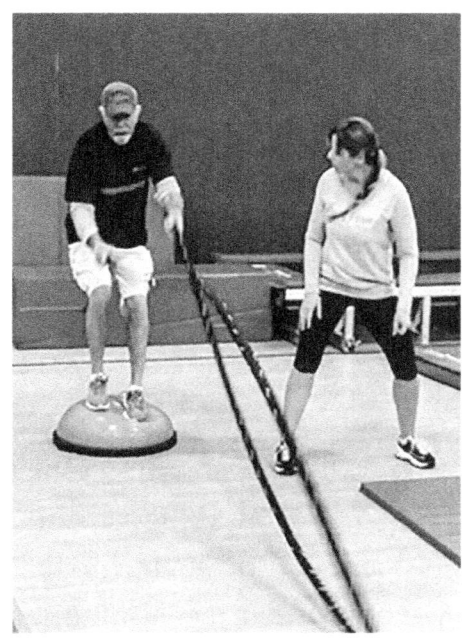

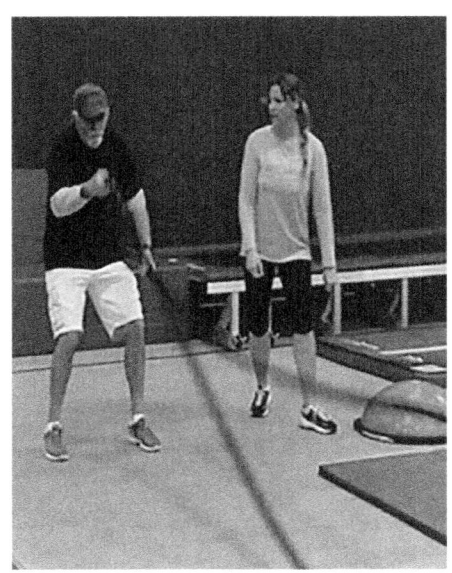

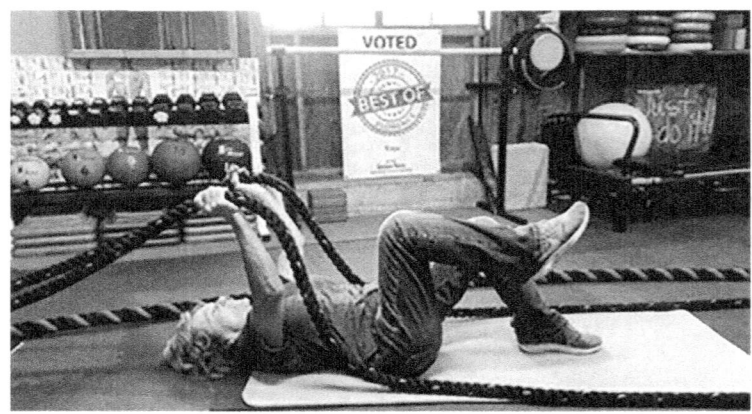

Combining battle ropes with some Pilates ab exercises is also a great source if the survivor's arms or shoulders can do it. In this exercise, the ropes are wrapped securely around a pole. This client is keeping the shoulders in place, and her abs are engaged as she slowly lifts one leg and lowers it back down with control while moving at the same speed both directions. She then rotates the right and the left leg with control. Combining this exercise with the ropes is a more advanced way of strengthening the core, arms, and shoulder stabilization. These are 30-pound, 30-foot ropes. They come in different lengths, diameters, and weights.

The ropes are usually fun for the clients. Many exercises can be done with them. It is something they can purchase and use at home once they can use them safely and know how to avoid injury using them on their own. They are excellent for neuro, cardio, and full-body workouts.

Here are some Exercises for the glutes and legs.

If you are unable to go to the floor safely or hold in these positions, do not do the floor exercises. Do the standing one holding onto a bar.

This first illustration is a standing exercise that exercises the glutes and some hip rotation muscles.

- Stand at the bar, as seen in the illustration.
- Stand tall, good posture, and engage your abs and your glutes engaged.
- Turn one foot slightly on an angle, as seen in the illustration.
- Lift and lower the leg, as seen in the illustration.

- Lift the leg by leading with the glutes, NOT your foot.

- This should be a controlled movement. Lifting the leg and lowering the leg with control. Control the movement in both directions. It is NOT a kicking up the leg and drops the leg exercise. Focus on lifting and lowering the leg.

- As you try to control the movements, it can be challenging. This is common.

- This standing exercise can be included with the floor exercise for those who can do both.

- It is okay to just do this standing exercise if you are unable to go to the floor. Remember, **Safety First!**

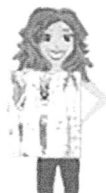 ***Reminders and tips.***

In time with practice, repetitiveness, and being consistent with movements, the body has a chance to master exercise movements and build the new pathways needed. As you gain back movements in exercises, this transfers over to everyday life movements and activities.

Don't give up!

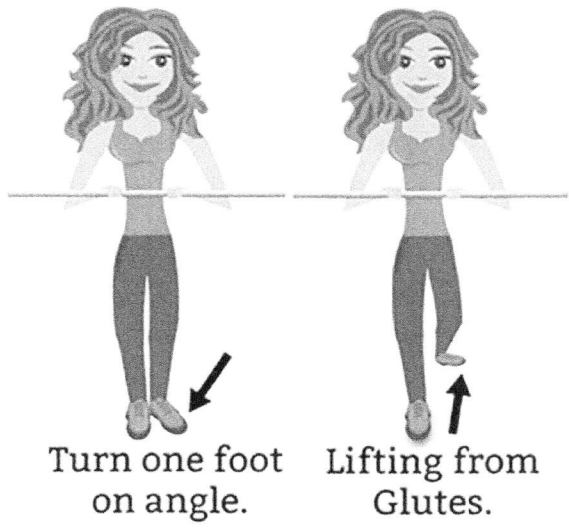

Turn one foot on angle.   Lifting from Glutes.

I call the next exercise the *Bent Leg Lift*. Proper positioning is important. Think of your body as a table, and all four table legs need to come straight down out of the corners of the tabletop. In this position, your knees should be under your hips and the elbows under your shoulders, as demonstrated in the following pictures with the checkmark. I understand some stroke survivors can do floor exercises, and others can not. Only do the exercises that may pertain to you at each step in your progress.

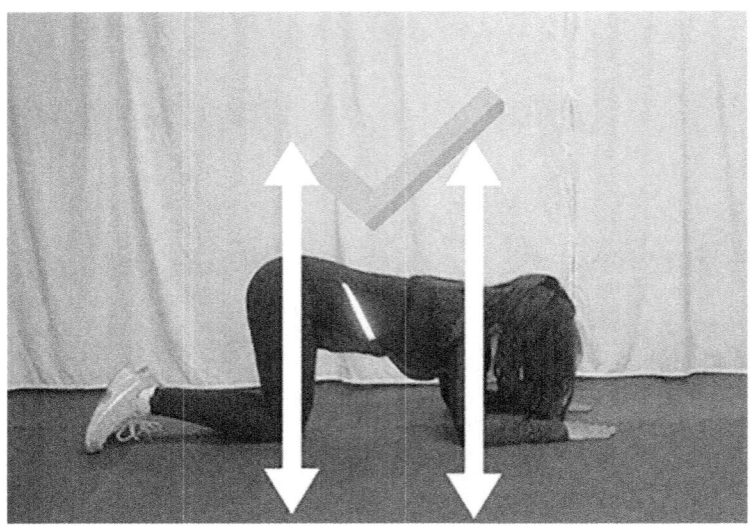

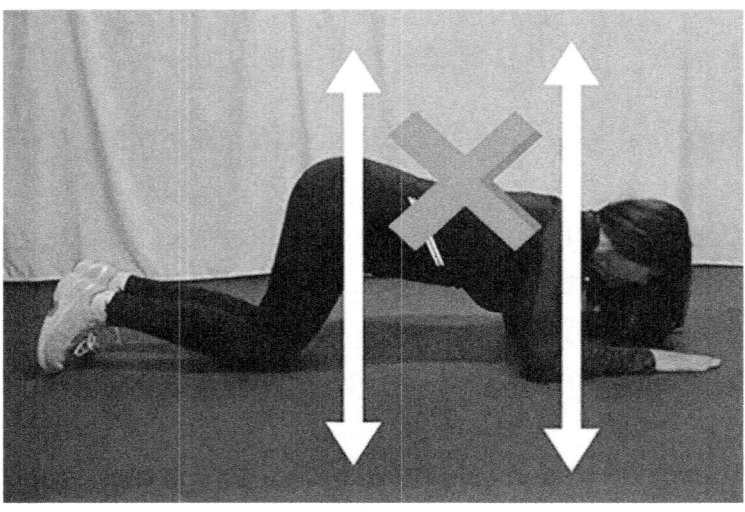

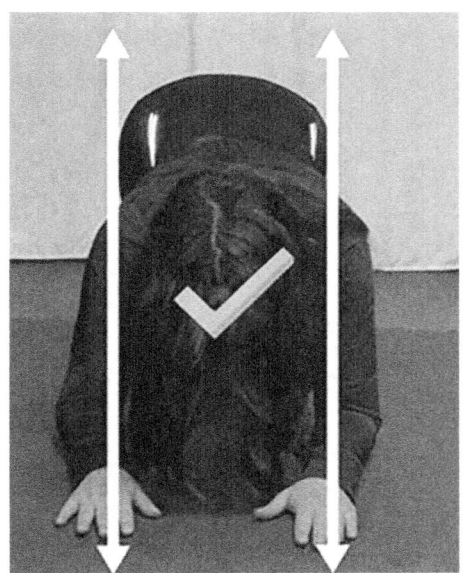

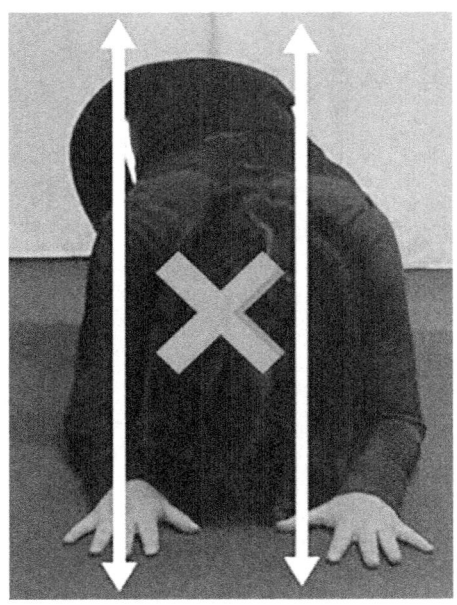

Once you are in the proper position, lift and lower the leg.

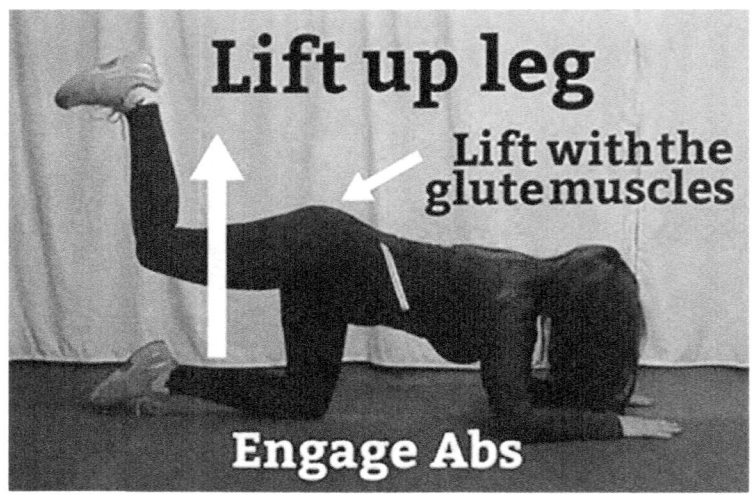

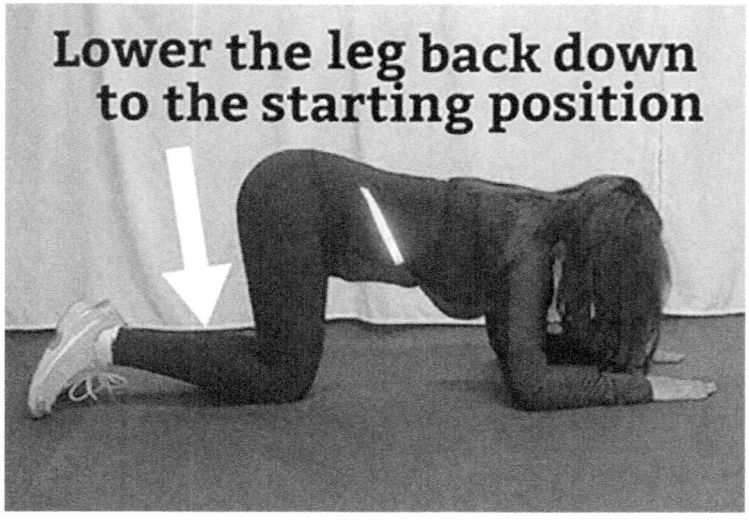

Another exercise that can be performed in the same positioning is the *straight leg, leg lift*. **This requires the same positioning as the previous bent leg, leg lift.**

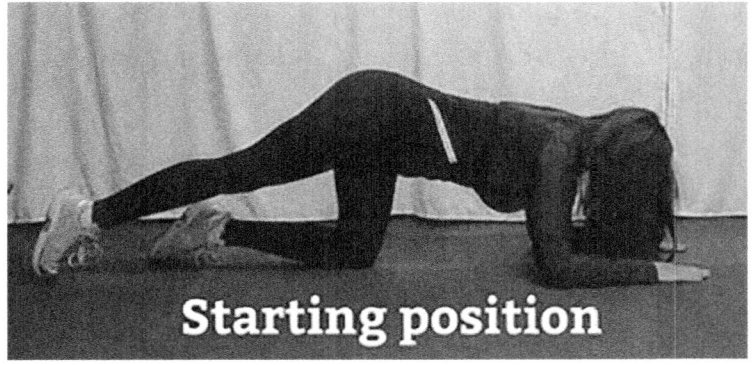

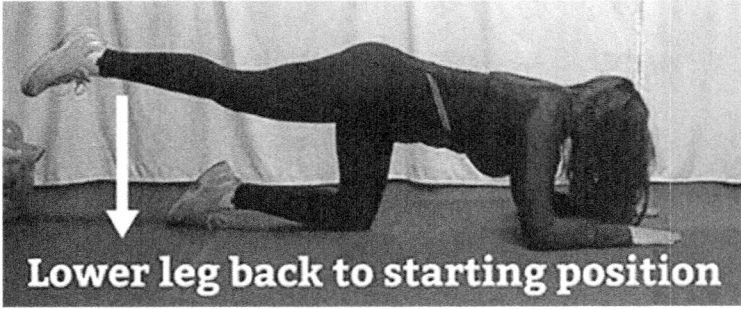

Both of these floor glute and leg exercises may be incredibly challenging for many at first. If you feel safe and can keep working on these, they can help build core stabilization, hip, and pelvic stabilization, shoulder stability, posture, spatial awareness, and proprioception. Many muscles are working together to keep the body in proper alignment. These exercises help to build the muscles and pathways needed for many everyday activities. They also help to train the muscles in the body to multitask again. The muscles have to relearn to work together subconsciously like they did before the stroke or weakness developed.

As with all exercise, I keep repeating, **only do the exercises that work at your level of recovery.**

Safety First!

Summing up the Exercises

Stroke recovery is complex and a tough, long journey for many survivors. As I mentioned previously in this book and my other books, not all exercises are for everyone. I include in my books and videos some of the exercises that I feel are important. You may have others that your therapist gave you to do, and if they are working, continue with them too. My books and knowledge are to add to what you may already know or not know.

You may have noticed that I did not say how many repetitions of each exercise to do. This is because that number is determined per individual case and recovery level. You may be able to do 5 squats holding the bar and be tired where another person may do 20 squats. It is all based on your strength in your recovery at that moment. You will have strong days and weaker days. That is normal. Do what you can that meets your level of energy for the day.

Please be patient with yourself if some exercise takes longer to master. That is normal. Each survivor has different muscles that need to come back into strength and movements. In some cases, parts of the body just do not come back, but there is a chance if you have more knowledge and do purposeful exercises that change can happen.

I like to say that a stroke recovery journey is like an athlete training for their sport. They think, sleep, and eat training. Physical recovery needs to be challenged every day. If you just do therapy exercise or practice standing up a couple of times a week and not several times a day (if possible), your recovery will be limited. Remember when babies learn to walk. They are trying to walk all day long when they can. They do not just try to walk once or twice a week.

I feel mat Pilates, and Pilates reformer exercises are a great addition in recovery as well.

Feed and nourish your brain and body with healthy foods and stay hydrated. The brain and body need to stay hydrated. It is essential.

My books *Stroke Recovery, What Now? When Physical Therapy Ends, but Your Recovery Continues* and *Stroke Recovery, Regaining Arm Movement* are great companions to this book.

I wish you a stronger recovery.

CHAPTER TEN

ABOUT THE AUTHOR

Tracy L. Markley has been working and studying in the fitness industry for over 20 years. She is the owner of Tracy's Personal Training, Pilates, and Yoga Studio. Previously in Huntington Beach, California, for 17 years and relocated to Oregon in 2013. Tracy is the radio show host of *The Health and Fitness Show with Tracy* on KXCR, 90.7 FM radio on the Oregon Coast. The show can also be heard worldwide on Twitch. Link to hear her radio show can be found at her websites. She is a Certified Health and Fitness Specialist, Personal Trainer, Dance & Group Exercise Leader, Fitness & Nutrition, Biomechanics Specialist, AFAA Group Exercise Examiner, BOSU® Master Trainer, FiTOUR Pro-Trainer, Reiki Master-Teacher, as well as a Pilates and Yoga Instructor. Her books and videos have helped stroke survivors and caregivers worldwide. In November 2017, she

published her first book, *The Stroke of an Artist"
The Journey of a Fitness Trainer and a Stroke
Survivor.* An inspiring journey of a stroke
survivor. In March 2018, she published her
second book, *Tipping Toward Balance," A
Fitness Trainer's Guide to Stability and Walking.*
This book is an excellent balance and fall
prevention book for all ages, including seniors.
Her third book, *Stroke Recovery What now? When
Physical Therapy Ends, But Recovery Continues*,
published in December 2018. Her fourth book,
*The Power of Your Spine, How Back Strength and
Posture Pilots the Entire Body*, was published in
September 2019. This book is also an Anatomy
Book. Her fifth book, *Stroke Recovery Regaining
Arm Movement,* published April 2020, Her sixth
book, *Dear Stroke You Suck, The Journey of A
Fitness Trainer and Stroke Survivor* is the
Original book *The Stroke of An Artist* republished
with a new book title, larger print and updated and
larger Anatomy Illustrations. Her seventh book,
*Stroke Recovery Leg Stability and Walking G*ait
and Her eighth book will be "*Your Brain*" The
Software of Your Body, A Fitness Trainer's
Guide to Brain Health. She is currently writing a

book on hearing loss since she grew up with a severe hearing loss.

In July 2018, she was asked to be on the Fitness Education Advisory Board for Medfited.org and to write CEC Certification Programs for professionals on Stroke Recovery and Exercise. She was awarded the 2019 Medical Fitness Professional of the Year First Runner up. In 2020 she was one of the three finalists for the IDEA Fitness Personal Trainer of the Year Award. Tracy is available for speaking events, book signings, and training. She can be contacted at her websites www.tracyspersonaltraining.com and www.tracymarkley.com

www.instagram.com/motivate_healthyfit
www.facebook.com/tracyfitt

YouTube Channel: Tracy L. Markley Fitness

Tracy's Books can be purchased
at her websites or Amazon at
www.amazon.com/author/tracymarkley

Author website www.tracymarkley.com

www.twitter.com/TracysFitnessHB

Tracy L. Markey is also the author of the following books:

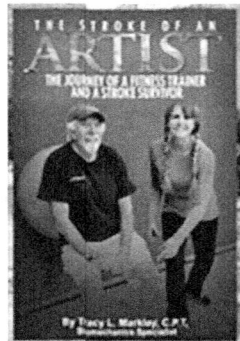
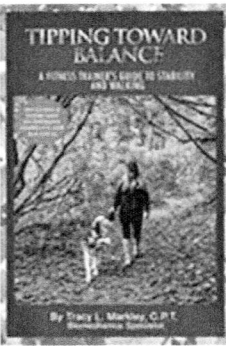
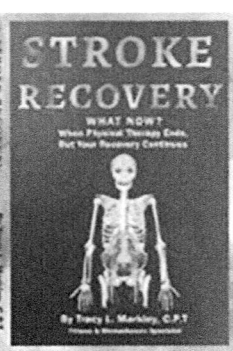

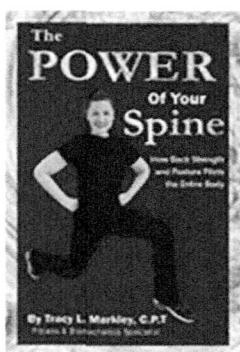
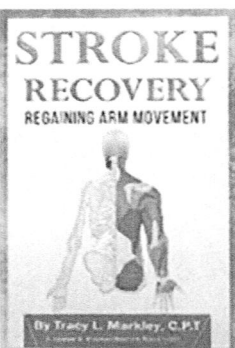
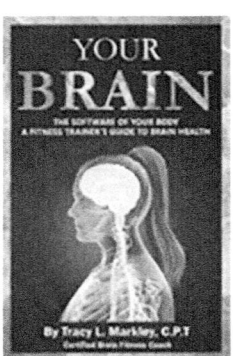

Books are available through Amazon at
www.amazon.com/author/tracymarkley

And her websites www.tracymarkley.com and
www.tracyspersonatraining.com

and www.strokerecoverybooks.com

REFERENCES

The Extremities by Quiring-Warfel

Kinesiology for the Public Schools, by J.A. Mastropaolo

The Power of Your Spine, by Tracy Markley

Stroke Recovery, What Now, by Tracy Markley

Albinus On Anatomy by Robert Beverly Hale and Terence Coyle

Years of schooling in Exercise and Biomechanics of the Human Body

REMEMBER,

PROPER

POSTURE

IS

ESSENTIAL

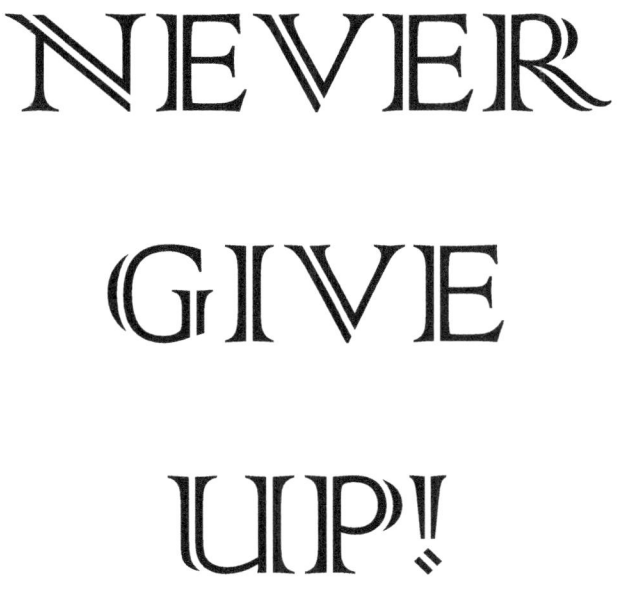

NEVER GIVE UP!

www.tracymarkley.com

www.strokerecoverybooks.com

www.tracyspersonaltraining.com

www.amazon.com/author/tracymarkley

Printed in Great Britain
by Amazon

23334360R00116